Mayo Clinic on Managing Incontinence

Paul Pettit, M.D.

Editor in Chief

Mayo Clinic
Rochester, Minnesota

Mayo Clinic on Managing Incontinence provides reliable information about getting help for incontinence. Much of the information comes directly from the experience of health care professionals at Mayo Clinic. This book supplements the advice of your personal physician, whom you should consult for individual medical problems. *Mayo Clinic on Managing Incontinence* does not endorse any company or product. MAYO, MAYO CLINIC, MAYO CLINIC HEALTH INFORMATION and the Mayo triple-shield logo are marks of Mayo Foundation for Medical Education and Research.

Published by Mayo Clinic Health Information, Rochester, Minn. Distributed to the book trade by Kensington Publishing Corporation, New York, N.Y. For bulk sales to employers, member groups and health-related companies, contact Mayo Clinic Health Management Resources, 200 First St. S.W., Rochester, MN 55905, or send e-mail to SpecialSalesMayoBooks@Mayo.edu.

Photo credits: Cover photos and the photos on pages 60, 99 and 133 are from PhotoDisc®; photos on pages vi and 1 are from Stockbyte.

Library of Congress Catalog Card Number: 2005921650

ISBN 1-893005-31-3

Printed in the United States of America

First Edition

1 2 3 4 5 6 7 8 9 10

About incontinence

Incontinence isn't something that's easy to talk about — especially when you or a loved one experiences it. Talking about it, whether with family and friends or with your doctor, takes courage. And discussing it is often the first step in getting help.

It has long been thought that incontinence was often just a result of the aging process, and there wasn't much that anyone could do to reduce or eliminate its effects. That's no longer true.

Significant advances have been made in the treatment of incontinence. New medications that reduce or eliminate the signs and symptoms of urinary incontinence are now available. Minimally invasive treatments with such materials as longer-lasting bulking agents offer relief to people with urinary incontinence. And developments in medical technology, such as sacral nerve stimulation, provide options for reducing or alleviating problems associated with both urinary and fecal incontinence.

Incontinence need not be something that you simply learn to live with. It can be treated, and in many cases improved or cured.

About Mayo Clinic

Mayo Clinic evolved from the frontier practice of Dr. William Worrall Mayo and the partnership of his two sons, William J. and Charles H. Mayo, in the early 1900s. Pressed by the demands of their busy practice in Rochester, Minn., the Mayo brothers invited other physicians to join them, pioneering the private group practice of medicine. Today, with more than 2,000 physicians and scientists at its three major locations in Rochester, Minn., Jacksonville, Fla., and Scottsdale, Ariz., Mayo Clinic is dedicated to providing comprehensive diagnoses, accurate answers and effective treatments.

With this depth of medical knowledge, experience and expertise, Mayo Clinic occupies an unparalleled position as a health information resource. Since 1983, Mayo Clinic has published reliable health information for millions of consumers through award-winning newsletters, books and online services. Revenue from the publishing activities supports Mayo Clinic programs, including medical education and research.

Editorial staff

Editor in Chief
Paul Pettit, M.D.

Managing Editor
Richard Dietman

Publisher
Sara Gilliland

Editor in Chief, Books and Newsletters
Christopher Frye

Copy Editor
Mary Duerson

Proofreading
Miranda Attlesey
Donna Hanson

Research Manager
Deirdre Herman

Research Librarians
Anthony Cook
Dana Gerberi
Michelle Hewlett

Contributing Writers
Rachel Bartony
Lee Engfer
Kelly Kershner

Creative Director
Daniel Brevick

Art Director
Stewart Koski

Illustration
Christopher Srnka

Medical Illustration
M. Alice McKinney

Indexing
Steve Rath

Administrative Assistants
Beverly Steele
Terri Zanto-Strausbauch

Contributing editors and reviewers

Anita Chen, M.D.
Heidi Chua, M.D.
Jeffrey Cornella, M.D.
Cynthia Feldt, M.P.T., A.T.C.
John Gebhart, M.D.
Nancy Itano, M.D.
Christopher Klingele, M.D.

Stephen Kramer, M.D.
Deborah Lightner, M.D.
John Pemberton, M.D.
Steven Petrou, M.D.
Mark Schwartz, Ph.D.
Karen Wallevand

iv

Preface

This book is intended to be a source of hope for all women, men and children who experience bladder and bowel control problems. Between 13 million and 20 million people in the United States have urinary incontinence, and more than 6 million people experience some form of fecal incontinence. Because of the assumed stigma, many people remain reluctant to talk about bladder and bowel problems with their doctors. Furthermore, many care providers still believe incontinence is a normal part of aging and that you need to just accept the problem and learn to live with it.

Our message is that most incontinence, whether bladder or bowel, can be improved or cured. Except for rare circumstances, therapy initially involves nonsurgical measures, such as changes in diet, bowel management, fluid control, physical therapy, Kegel exercises and either the elimination or addition of medications. If these approaches don't give you the quality of life you desire, or the medications can't be tolerated, then measures such as surgery may be an option.

This book can help you select a care provider and prepare for an office visit. It describes testing that may be needed to diagnose your specific type of incontinence, and it explains the numerous therapy options that are available. We've also included an appendix for quick reference to items such as dietary restrictions, Kegel exercises, bladder drills, medications that can cause or worsen incontinence, and Internet references to other resources. We hope this book helps you gain a better understanding of incontinence, and that it serves as a guide to getting effective medical care that leads to a better quality of life.

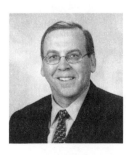

Paul Pettit, M.D.
Editor in Chief

Contents

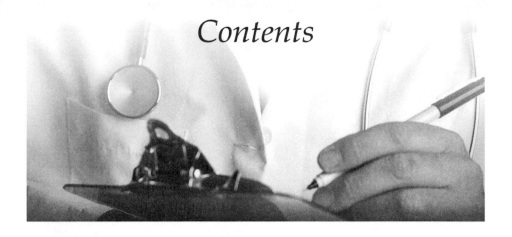

Part 2: Fecal Incontinence

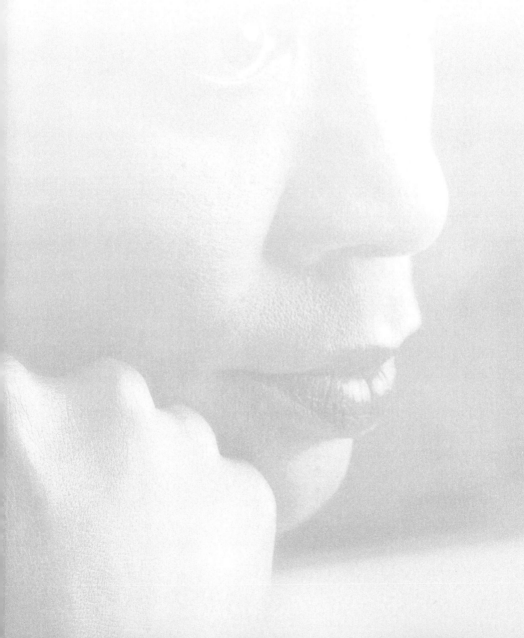

Part 1

Urinary incontinence

Chapter 1

Do you have urinary incontinence?

While on your way to the shopping mall, do you review in your mind the exact location of each and every bathroom before you get there? When you're out having fun with friends, do you consciously suppress laughing for fear of wetting yourself? As you insert the key into the lock on the door to your house or apartment, are you overwhelmed by an uncontrollable urge to urinate? Do you leak urine when you cough or sneeze?

If you answered yes to any of these questions, you may have urinary incontinence — the inability to hold urine until you can get to a bathroom. You may experience only occasional, minor leaks or dribbles of urine. Or your problem may be so severe that you wet yourself frequently. Urinary incontinence is generally defined as the involuntary loss of urine that's severe enough to be a social or personal hygiene problem. Doctors generally provide a diagnosis of urinary incontinence when urine leakage is sufficient enough to have a negative effect on your quality of life, especially in social situations.

Urinary incontinence is a medical condition

Here's the truth. Urinary incontinence isn't a normal part of childbearing or aging. It has many causes, some relatively simple and temporary and others more involved and long term. And although it's a medical condition, urinary incontinence can also affect other aspects of your life, including your finances and psychological well-being.

Urinary incontinence can be treated, and in many cases, it can be eliminated entirely. Even when it can't be completely eliminated, proper treatment can ease the discomfort and inconvenience of incontinence and improve your quality of life. And with today's medical advances, most people with urinary incontinence can be helped in some way.

An estimated $20 billion a year is spent in the United States to treat and manage urinary incontinence. Most of this money goes toward absorbent pads and other products for managing the condition. About 10 percent of it goes toward diagnosis and treatment. If you've been struggling with urinary incontinence, you may know all too well how the condition can affect your pocketbook.

Urinary incontinence can also take an emotional toll. Embarrassment associated with the condition can lead to social withdrawal, depression, anxiety and even sexual dysfunction. One study found that women with severe urinary incontinence were 80 percent more likely to experience significant depression, compared with women who weren't incontinent. In another study, researchers found that men and women with urinary incontinence had a 50 percent higher risk of having symptoms of anxiety, compared with men and women who didn't have incontinence.

If you're having a problem with urinary incontinence, you may be reluctant to talk with your doctor about it. Studies suggest that at least half of the people struggling with urinary incontinence don't report the problem to their doctors or other health care professionals. You may be embarrassed to talk about it, as many people are. Or you may have convinced yourself that urinary incontinence is something you just have to learn to live with. You may believe the common misconception that urinary incontinence is an inevitable consequence of childbearing, menopause or just growing older — and that it's a waste of time to try to do anything about it. Even some doctors take this view.

If you're having trouble with urinary incontinence, don't let embarrassment get the better of you. See your doctor. If he or she doesn't have a positive attitude about treating incontinence, then seek another care provider, perhaps someone who specializes in treating incontinence. Although urinary incontinence isn't a disease, it often indicates an underlying condition that likely can be treated. A thorough evaluation by your doctor can help determine what's behind your incontinence. Once you've made that important first step to get an evaluation, you'll be well on your way to regaining a more active and confident life.

How common is urinary incontinence?

The inability to control the release of urine from your bladder — urinary incontinence — is common. Estimates vary, but most experts put the number of Americans affected by the condition at between 13 million and 20 million.

Urinary incontinence is much more common among women than men. Among women ages 15 to 64, it's estimated that between 10 percent and 30 percent have urinary incontinence. Among men in this same age range, the estimated prevalence is much lower — just 1 percent to 5 percent.

What accounts for the difference? A woman's urethra — the tube that runs from the bladder to the urethral opening — is much shorter than a man's (see the illustration on page 7). That means a woman's urine has a shorter distance to travel to cause leakage. Other possible reasons for the difference are pregnancy and childbirth, which can weaken or damage the pelvic floor muscles and the ring of muscles that surrounds the urethra, that is, the urethral sphincter (u-REE-thrahl SFINGK-tur). With these muscles weakened, urine may escape whenever pressure is placed on the bladder.

Another reason for the difference is menopause. The drop in estrogen that follows menopause affects the organs and tissues of the lower urinary tract. It can contribute to changes in the linings of the bladder and the urethra, making them less elastic and able to stay closed. After menopause a woman's urethral sphincter may simply not be able to hold in urine as easily as it did before, leading to urinary incontinence.

In men, incontinence is more closely associated with aging and aging-related health problems. Among men older than age 60 who are living at home, between 5 percent and 15 percent have urinary incontinence. Prostate disease is also a significant factor. An enlarged prostate gland (benign prostatic hyperplasia), prostate surgery and other treatments for prostate cancer can all cause degrees of urinary incontinence in men.

Urinary incontinence is not a "normal" part of aging. That said, however, the problem does increase with age. Doctors and scientists estimate that among adults age 65 and older who are still living in their homes, 15 percent to 30 percent have urinary incontinence. When you consider those living in long term care facilities, the number climbs to at least 50 percent.

Why is this? As you get older, the muscles in your bladder and urethra lose some of their strength. These age-related changes reduce the amount of urine your bladder can hold, which means you have to urinate more often. If you don't heed the call promptly enough, urinary incontinence can result.

With age your pelvic floor muscles also can become weaker, further compromising your ability to hold urine. Some research suggests that your bladder muscle (detrusor) becomes overactive with age. An overactive bladder muscle creates the urge to urinate before your bladder is full, which can lead to urinary incontinence.

The bottom line? Millions of people experience urinary incontinence every day. Men and women of all ages are affected, some more than others. The good news is that it's treatable — and often curable — at all ages, for both men and women.

Understanding your urinary system

To understand urinary incontinence, it helps to have some basic knowledge about the organs and other structures that make the urinary system work. When you eat and drink, your body breaks down what you eat and drink into substances that can be absorbed into your bloodstream. Your body absorbs liquid and nutrients, but excess fluid and waste accumulate in your bloodstream. The job of your urinary system is to remove, collect, store and eliminate these waste products from your bloodstream — and ultimately from your body — through the process of urination.

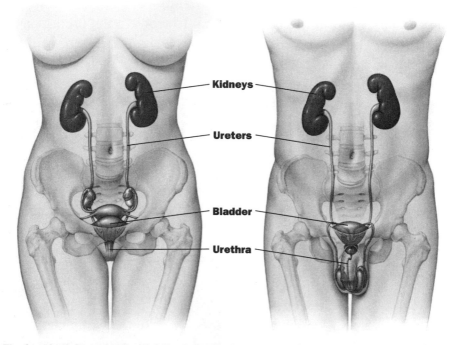

The female (left) and male (right) urinary tracts are essentially the same. The main difference is that in women, the urethra is shorter than in men.

Upper urinary system

Your urinary system has two main parts — upper and lower. The upper urinary system consists of two kidneys, each attached to a long, muscular tube, called a ureter (u-REE-tur).

The kidneys are your body's primary filtration system, removing excess fluid and waste from your bloodstream to make urine. Adult-size kidneys filter about 42 gallons of blood each day and make about 1 1/2 quarts of urine. The ureters carry this urine to the bladder, delivering it continuously in small, steady amounts. Gravity and muscle contractions in the ureters force the urine through the ureters to the bladder.

Lower urinary tract

Your lower urinary tract consists of the bladder, a slender drainage tube at its base called the urethra (u-REE-thrah), and two ring-like bands of muscles at the junction of the bladder and urethra called the internal and external urethral sphincters.

The bladder — a muscular, balloon-like sac — stores urine. When you urinate, the bladder muscle contracts, pushing urine out of the bladder and through the urethra. In women, the urethra is about $1^1/_2$ inches long, and its opening to the outside of the body is located just above the vagina, between the clitoris and the vaginal opening. In men the urethra is about 8 inches long. It passes through the walnut-shaped prostate gland at the base of the bladder and through the entire length of the penis. Its opening is at the tip of the penis.

The urethral sphincters help control the release of urine. The internal sphincter, made up of muscles over which you have no control (involuntary muscles), keeps your urethra closed while your bladder is filling, preventing urine from leaking out. This happens with no conscious effort on your part. When your bladder is nearly full, the internal sphincter automatically relaxes, responding to a message from the bladder control center of the brain. That's when the external sphincter goes to work. Made up of muscles you can consciously control (voluntary muscles), the external sphincter counters the relaxing action of the internal sphincter, helping you keep the urethra closed until you can get to the bathroom to urinate.

Playing a supporting role in all of this are the pelvic floor muscles — which make up a hammock-like network of muscles that extends from your pubic bone, in the front of your pelvis, to your tailbone, at the base of your spine. When you urinate, the pelvic floor muscles relax, allowing urine to pass out of your body easily. Between episodes of urination, the pelvic floor muscles lightly contract, holding in urine and supporting your bladder from underneath. Nerves that run from the spinal cord to the bladder coordinate the action of the pelvic floor muscles. Because these muscles are under voluntary control, they can be strengthened with exercise (see "Pelvic floor exercises" in the Appendix on page 191).

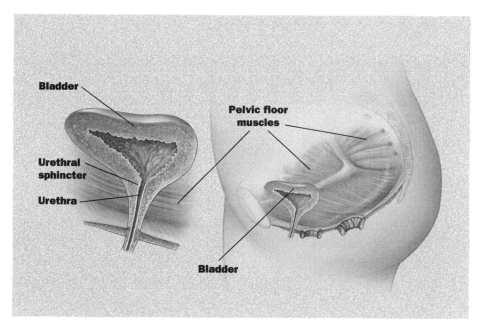

Bladder

Pelvic floor muscles

Urethral sphincter

Urethra

Bladder

Your pelvic floor muscles stretch across the pelvis and support structures of the lower abdomen, including the bladder. When pelvic floor muscles become weakened, incontinence may result.

Normal urination

Normal urination is a coordinated process involving the many organs, tubes, muscles and nerves in your urinary system. Once the bladder is nearly full, nerves there send a signal to the brain. The brain then sends a message to relax the internal urethral sphincter, creating the first urge to urinate. You then decide whether it's the appropriate time and place to do so.

When you decide to urinate, several things happen. The external urethral sphincter and pelvic floor muscles relax, allowing urine to pass out of your body. The internal urethral sphincter also relaxes, increasing pressure inside the bladder and pushing urine into the urethra. Then the bladder muscle contracts, and urine passes through the urethra and out of your body.

Good bladder control isn't as simple as it may seem. Urination is a complex process that involves relaxing part of your pelvis while contracting another part. The organs, tubes, muscles and nerves in your urinary system must work together. If any part malfunctions, incontinence can result.

Types of urinary incontinence

Urinary incontinence — the inability to control the release of urine from your bladder — is classified by your signs and symptoms or the circumstances at the time you leak urine. The five main types are stress incontinence, overactive bladder, mixed incontinence, overflow incontinence and functional incontinence.

Stress incontinence

Stress incontinence refers to leaking urine when you exert pressure on your bladder by coughing, sneezing, laughing, exercising or lifting something heavy. The leakage occurs even though your bladder muscle is not contracting, and you may not feel the urge to urinate. The problem is especially noticeable when your bladder becomes too full. Coughing, laughing or exerting yourself may cause a little urine to seep out or may even cause a larger squirt.

Stress incontinence can be quite upsetting, but the condition has nothing to do with psychological stress. Used here, the word *stress* refers to the physical strain on your bladder that occurs because of actions that increase pressure in your abdomen.

Doctors typically classify stress incontinence into two subtypes — urethral hypermobility and intrinsic sphincteric deficiency.

Overflow	Stress	Overactive bladder
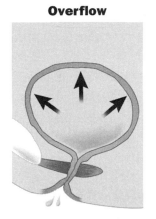	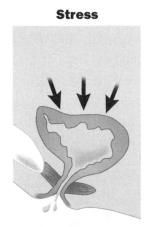	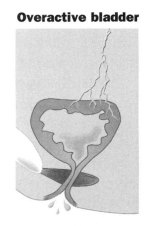

Overflow incontinence (left) is characterized by frequent urination or dribbling of urine. In stress incontinence (center), urine leaks when you exert pressure on your bladder when coughing, laughing, lifting, or simply getting out of bed. With overactive bladder (right), your bladder muscle contracts too often, signaling your brain that you have to urinate. it's characterized by a sudden, involuntary loss of bladder control.

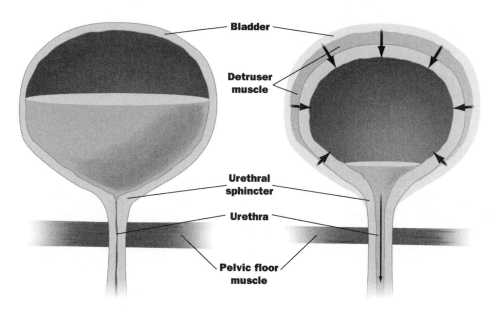

The detrusor muscle surrounds the bladder. When it contracts (right), and when the urethral sphincter at the base of the bladder relaxes, urine flows through the urethra.

- With urethral hypermobility, the bladder and urethra shift downward in response to increased abdominal pressure, and there isn't enough support from the hammock-like pelvic floor muscles to help keep the urethra closed. As a result, urine leaks out when you cough, laugh or sneeze.
- With intrinsic sphincteric deficiency, there's a problem with your sphincter that keeps it from closing completely or allows it to open under pressure, leaving your urethra open like a drainpipe. This, too, causes urine to leak out when you cough, laugh, sneeze or otherwise increase the pressure in your abdomen.

In women, stress incontinence may be a result of pelvic floor muscles and nerves that have been weakened or damaged during pregnancy and childbirth. Some experts believe that women who've delivered vaginally are at highest risk of developing stress incontinence, although not all studies support this view. Aging and decreased estrogen with menopause are known factors. In men, the most common cause of stress incontinence is damage to the urethral sphincter sustained as a result of prostate surgery or a broken hip.

Men and women who have lung conditions that cause frequent coughing, such as emphysema, often develop stress incontinence. Frequent coughing puts stress on your urinary sphincter. Longtime smokers also experience stress incontinence for this reason.

Overactive bladder

Overactive bladder is most often characterized by a frequent urge to urinate, sometimes followed by a sudden and involuntary loss of bladder control before you can reach a bathroom. Normally, you urinate six or seven times a day, with your bladder holding 6 to 12 ounces of urine. With overactive bladder, you may urinate 13 or more times a day, all in small amounts. The urge to urinate may even wake you up several times a night. Urinating this often is called urinary frequency. Awakening at night to urinate is called nocturia.

An important symptom of overactive bladder is urinary urgency — the strong, sudden need to urinate immediately. Your body may give you a warning of only a few seconds to a minute to reach a toilet.

With overactive bladder, your bladder muscle contracts too often and at inappropriate times — namely, when your bladder isn't full. Your brain then gets the message that you have to go — now.

When you leak urine as the result of an overactive bladder, it's called urge incontinence. You may leak or gush urine as the result of a sudden, intense urge to urinate. Some people with urge incontinence leak urine when they hear running water or after they drink only a small amount of liquid. Putting your hands under running water to wash dishes may even cause you to leak urine.

Another common problem is called key-in-the-lock syndrome or garage door syndrome. Because you associate arriving home with being able to urinate, you may feel an overwhelming urge to urinate and leak urine — literally as you put your key in the lock or open the garage door.

Urge incontinence may be caused by a urinary tract infection or by something that irritates the bladder. It can also be caused by bowel problems or damage to the nervous system associated with multiple sclerosis, diabetes, Parkinson's disease, Alzheimer's disease, stroke, or injury to the brain, spine or nerves extending from the spine to the bladder — including injury that inadvertently occurs during surgery. In many cases the cause of overactive bladder and urge incontinence isn't known.

In women, urge incontinence typically occurs after menopause, perhaps as a result of changes in the bladder lining and muscle caused by decreased estrogen. In men, urge incontinence can be the result of a prostate infection, an enlarged prostate (benign prostatic hyperplasia), or freezing (cryotherapy) or radiation seed treatment (brachytherapy) for prostate cancer.

Mixed incontinence

Mixed incontinence means having more than one type of incontinence, typically stress incontinence and urge incontinence. You have signs and symptoms of both types. You leak urine when you cough, laugh, sneeze or otherwise increase the pressure in your abdomen — signaling stress incontinence. And you also have accidents in which you have a strong urge to urinate but can't reach the toilet in time — signaling urge incontinence. With mixed incontinence, one type is typically more bothersome than the other is. The cause of the two forms may or may not be related.

The combination of stress incontinence and urge incontinence often occurs in women. In fact, some experts say that most women with urinary incontinence have signs and symptoms of both stress and urge incontinence. But mixed incontinence is not exclusively a women's problem. Men who've had their prostate glands removed or who've had surgery for enlarged prostates can develop mixed incontinence. Older adults also often experience a combination of stress and urge incontinence.

Overflow incontinence

With overflow incontinence, you frequently or even constantly dribble small amounts of urine throughout the day. You may feel as if you never completely empty your bladder — or that you need to empty your bladder but can't. When you try to urinate, you may have trouble getting started and may produce only a weak stream of urine. When urine leaks out, you may or may not have felt the urge to urinate.

Overflow incontinence stems from the inability to completely empty your bladder. Over time, urine accumulates until it exceeds your bladder's capacity to hold it. The increased pressure at the base of your bladder becomes too much to bear. The pressure forces your urethral sphincter to open, and the overflow urine leaks out.

Incomplete or poor bladder emptying can occur if your urethra is blocked in some way, obstructing urine from flowing normally out of your bladder. It can also be the result of weak or underactive bladder muscles that don't contract forcefully enough or often enough to empty the bladder and maintain normal urination. Think of this as the opposite of urge incontinence caused by an overactive bladder.

Overflow incontinence is common among men with prostate gland problems. An enlarged prostate gland can surround and narrow or block the urethra, preventing the bladder from emptying. Tumors, bladder stones and scar tissue also can block the urethra, keeping urine from leaving the bladder normally.

Nerve damage from diabetes, multiple sclerosis, shingles, injury or other diseases also can lead to overflow incontinence. Damaged nerves can lead to weak bladder muscles, preventing them from contracting normally during urination. Medications that prevent your bladder from contracting normally or make you unaware of the urge to urinate can also cause or increase overflow incontinence. These may include painkillers, antidepressants and smooth muscle relaxants. (For a list of medications that may cause or worsen urinary incontinence, see pages 192-193.)

Overflow incontinence is fairly rare among women. However, it can occur as the result of nerve damage sustained during childbirth. Women with severe prolapse of the uterus or bladder also sometimes experience overflow incontinence. With the uterus or bladder sagging out of its proper position, the urethra can become kinked, interfering with the normal flow of urine.

If left untreated, overflow incontinence can have serious consequences. The urine retained in your bladder can become infected, and this infection may spread throughout the entire urinary tract. In severe cases urine can back up into the kidneys. Called reflux, this can damage the kidneys and affect kidney function.

Other types of urinary incontinence

You may hear a variety of terms to describe urinary incontinence. Reflex incontinence occurs among people with serious neurological impairment, such as those with the birth defect spina bifida or those with paralysis from a spinal cord injury that affects the nerves running to the bladder. Damage to these nerves prevents the transfer of messages between the brain and the bladder, leading to urine loss without any sensation or warning.

A fistula is an abnormal opening between the bladder and another structure, such as the vagina or rectum. This can cause a leak in the urinary system that also can cause incontinence.

Reversible incontinence is the term used to describe urine leakage that occurs temporarily because of a condition that will pass. It has many possible triggers, including urinary tract infection, mental impairment, restricted mobility and a severe form of constipation called stool impaction.

Total incontinence is a term that's sometimes used to describe continuous leaking of urine, day and night, or periodic large volumes of urine and uncontrollable leaking. Some people have this type of incontinence because they were born with a physical defect. It can also be caused by a spinal cord injury or by injury to the urinary system from surgery.

Nocturnal enuresis (en-u-REE-sis) is the medical term for nighttime bed-wetting. Some children, mainly boys, who are otherwise toilet trained wet the bed at night for a variety of reasons. Adults can lose control of their bladder at night, too, possibly because of alcohol or medications. The aging bladder also is more likely to have difficulty storing urine at night. That, coupled with the fact that the kidneys generally more readily filter and eliminate fluid when you're lying down, can lead to greater urine production during sleep.

Functional incontinence

Functional incontinence is the inability to make it to the toilet in time because of a physical or mental illness, impairment, or disability that's unrelated to your urinary system. For example, if you have severe arthritis in your hands, you may not be able to unbutton your pants quickly enough, and you may leak urine. If you're in a wheelchair or you have trouble walking, getting to a toilet quickly may be difficult. It may be hard for you to avoid accidents — even though your urinary system is functioning properly.

Many of the conditions that lead to functional incontinence are associated with aging. Dementia, including Alzheimer's disease, affects your ability to think about urinating. It can make you unaware of the need to find a toilet or can lead to confusion about where it is and how to use it.

Barriers in the home environment also sometimes play a role. Having a bathroom that's too far away — especially if it's upstairs and there are no handrails — can be a hindrance in getting to the bathroom in time. Sometimes, just the fear of falling is enough to prevent an older person from going upstairs to use the toilet.

Not surprisingly, many older adults in hospitals and nursing homes experience functional incontinence. Some experts estimate that more than 25 percent of the urinary incontinence occurring in hospitals and nursing homes is functional incontinence.

Medications can sometimes lead to functional incontinence. Diuretics used to treat high blood pressure or congestive heart failure can cause you to produce abnormally large amounts of urine. Some medications can decrease your awareness of the need to find a toilet. Functional incontinence that's triggered by medications is sometimes referred to as transient incontinence because changing or discontinuing the medication may solve the problem.

Reasons to hope

It's important to remember that, despite the embarrassment and social stigma associated with it, urinary incontinence is a medical condition that in many cases can be successfully treated. In the chapters ahead, you'll learn more details about the various types of incontinence, as well as information about behavior therapy, medications and surgery used to treat it. Remember, talking about urinary incontinence with a trusted care provider is often the first step in overcoming the problem.

Chapter 2

Causes of urinary incontinence

Doctors and scientists generally divide the causes of urinary incontinence into two categories — temporary and persistent. Persistent causes are underlying physical problems that usually can't be changed. Temporary — also called transient — causes can often be reversed with treatment or with lifestyle changes. For example, if you drink a lot of water or other beverages, particularly over a short period of time, you increase the amount of urine your bladder has to hold. This may result in an occasional wetting accident. On the other hand, if you don't drink enough to stay properly hydrated, your urine may become overly concentrated. The increased concentration of body salts can irritate your bladder and may lead to incontinence.

Consuming too much caffeine also can be a reversible cause of urinary incontinence. Caffeine is a diuretic. As such, it causes your bladder to fill more quickly than usual, resulting in an urgent and sometimes uncontrollable need to urinate. For some people, noncaffeinated carbonated drinks, teas and coffees irritate the bladder and may cause episodes of urinary incontinence. Citrus fruits and juices and artificial sweeteners also can be bladder irritants. (For more on bladder irritants, see page 188 of the Appendix.)

Persistent causes that may lead to urinary incontinence include aging, menopause, previous surgery, weakened muscles, nerve problems and a variety of medical conditions. When these factors are involved, urinary incontinence may be chronic and ongoing.

Even if its root cause can't be reversed, urinary incontinence can almost always be treated. Treatment depends on the type of incontinence, the severity of the problem and the underlying cause. In fact, most people who are treated for urinary incontinence see a dramatic improvement in their signs and symptoms.

Temporary causes of urinary incontinence

The reversible causes of incontinence can be remembered with the acronym DIAP(P)ERS — delirium, infection of the urinary tract, atrophic urethritis or vaginitis, pharmaceuticals, psychological problems, excessive urine output, restricted mobility and stool impaction. In addition, recent evidence supports the inclusion of two additional causes — being overweight and a lack of physical fitness. Here's a brief overview of each temporary cause of urinary incontinence.

Delirium
Delirium is defined as a severely confused mental state. Its causes include medications, sleep deprivation and acute illness, such as an infection or kidney or liver failure. Some people also become delirious in reaction to anesthesia. When you're delirious or confused, for whatever reason, you may temporarily lose bladder control. In this context, urinary incontinence is a symptom of an altered mental state. Once the underlying cause of confusion is identified and treated, the problem of incontinence generally goes away.

Consuming alcohol to excess also can cause confusion and urinary incontinence. If you drink too much, it may temporarily impair your ability to recognize the need to urinate — and to act on that need in a timely way.

Infection of the urinary tract
A urinary tract infection is an infection that begins in your urinary system, typically in your urethra or bladder, or both. A bladder infection is called cystitis. An infection of the urethra is known as

urethritis. Urinary tract infections typically occur when bacteria from the outside enter the urinary tract through the urethra and begin to multiply in the bladder. The resulting infection irritates your bladder, causing you to experience strong urges to urinate. These urges are sometimes so strong that you can't get to the bathroom in time, resulting in episodes of urinary incontinence. When you experience sudden or worsening urine leakage, doctors generally recommend having a simple urine test to rule out urinary tract infection as a cause.

It's possible to have bacteria in your urine and not have a urinary tract infection. Some people, especially older adults, may have bacteria in the bladder that don't cause any signs or symptoms or harm. This condition is known as asymptomatic bacteriuria, and it doesn't cause urinary incontinence. In general, urinary tract infections cause incontinence only when they are accompanied by other urinary signs and symptoms, such as a strong, persistent urge to urinate, foul-smelling urine or a burning sensation when urinating.

Urinary tract infection is a common cause of urinary incontinence, but it's easily reversible with treatment. If your symptoms are typical and you're generally in good health, antibiotics are the first line of treatment for most urinary tract infections. Usually, symptoms of a urinary tract infection, including urinary incontinence, clear up within a few days of treatment.

Atrophic urethritis or vaginitis

After menopause a woman's estrogen level falls dramatically. The decline in estrogen causes the tissues of the urethra and vagina to become drier, thinner, less elastic and more susceptible to irritation. This condition is known as atrophic urethritis or atrophic vaginitis, depending on where it occurs, and it can contribute to urinary incontinence.

Women who have atrophic urethritis or vaginitis typically report increased urinary frequency and urgency, sometimes resulting in urge incontinence. But the condition can also cause or contribute to stress incontinence. As the tissues of the urethra become thinner, they lose resistance. This can lead to urine leakage when your bladder contains urine and you're upright and active. If you also have weak pelvic floor and sphincter muscles, your risk of urine leakage may be especially high.

Atrophic urethritis or vaginitis may be treated with estrogen applied to the vaginal area, usually as a cream. Vaginal estrogen tablets and rings also are available. The estrogen, which helps to restore vaginal tissue, stays primarily in the vaginal area, although a small amount is absorbed into the bloodstream. Your doctor may prescribe a low-dose estrogen preparation daily for a month or two and then gradually taper it to just three or four times a month. Estrogen therapy in pill or patch form is less effective and poses additional risks, especially for women who have had breast or uterine cancer.

Pharmaceuticals
Medications are one of the most common causes of urinary incontinence. Sedatives, such as sleeping pills, can sometimes interfere with your ability to control bladder function. Other medications — including diuretics, muscle relaxants and antidepressants — can cause or increase incontinence. Some high blood pressure drugs, heart medications and cold medicines also can affect bladder function.

Because each type of medication affects your body in a different way, each has its own potential mechanism for causing incontinence. For a list of types of medications that may contribute to urinary incontinence, see page 192 of the Appendix.

Psychological problems
In rare cases, psychological problems, especially severe depression, may result in urinary incontinence. This may be especially true after major surgery or after being diagnosed with a serious illness. The resulting depression, which is not uncommon, may make you lose interest in all aspects of personal hygiene, including staying clean and dry.

It's sometimes hard to know, however, whether severe depression is directly to blame for urinary incontinence. If you're recovering from surgery or being treated for a serious illness, you may be taking medications that contribute to incontinence. More research is needed to pinpoint the exact role of psychological causes.

Excessive urine output

Producing an abnormally large amount of urine over a given period of time is known as polyuria. It can be a side effect of a medical problem, such as uncontrolled diabetes. Early signs of high blood sugar (hyperglycemia) are increased thirst and frequent urination. Excessive urine output can also be caused by disorders associated with fluid overload, such as congestive heart failure.

Medications can be another cause of polyuria, especially diuretics, theophylline and dihydropyridine calcium channel blockers. Drinking caffeinated beverages, alcohol or an excessive amount of water also can cause excessive urine output.

Polyuria is a common cause of urinary incontinence. If you're producing large amounts of urine, you may not be able to get to the bathroom quickly enough to prevent a wetting accident. When you have to get up several times a night to urinate — and you sometimes don't make it — excessive urine output may be to blame.

Treatment for polyuria involves controlling or correcting the underlying cause of the problem, whether it's a medication, a medical problem or excessive fluid intake. Once your polyuria is under control, the problem of urinary incontinence usually goes away on its own.

Restricted mobility

There are many reasons why people have a hard time getting around. Arthritis, hip pain or foot problems can make it difficult to walk. Other medical problems, such as congestive heart failure, can be so exhausting that walking more than a short distance is nearly impossible. Poor eyesight, injury, fear of falling and medication-induced confusion also can restrict your mobility.

If your mobility is restricted to the point that you can't respond promptly to the urge to urinate, urinary incontinence can result. If you're recovering from a stroke, you may not be able to walk quickly enough to reach the bathroom in time. If your joints are swollen because of severe arthritis, you may not have the dexterity necessary to undo your clothes in time to avoid leaking urine. Being confined to a hospital bed because of an acute illness or major surgery also can cause temporary incontinence. In general, the more difficult it is for you to move, the greater your likelihood of experiencing incontinence.

If you're having trouble getting around and you think it might be contributing to urinary incontinence, talk with your doctor. The underlying problem may be more treatable than you think it is.

Stool impaction

Chronic constipation may lead to impacted stool — a large mass of dry, hard stool within your rectum. The hard mass of stool puts pressure on your perineum — the area between the vulva and anus in women and between the scrotum and anus in men. This pressure, in turn, obstructs the flow of urine at the bottom (neck) of the bladder. Impacted stool typically results in an inability to empty the bladder, which can lead to overflow incontinence. But it also may cause increased contractions of the bladder muscle (detrusor) and episodes of urge incontinence. The theory is that because the rectum and bladder share many of the same nerves, unmoved stools in your rectum cause these nerves to be overactive, ultimately causing urine leakage.

Stool impaction is a relatively common cause of urinary incontinence. Doctors estimate that it's the direct cause of the problem in up to 10 percent of older adults admitted to the hospital for acute care or referred to incontinence clinics. Disimpacting the stool usually solves the problem of urinary incontinence. To remove an impacted stool, your doctor inserts one or two fingers into your rectum and breaks the impacted stool into fragments that you can later expel.

Being overweight

Obesity is a risk factor for urinary incontinence, especially among women. Being significantly overweight puts constant, increased pressure on your bladder and its surrounding muscles, nerves and other structures, weakening them and allowing urine to leak out when you cough or sneeze (stress incontinence). Obesity is also implicated as a factor in urge incontinence, although the relationship is not quite as strong. Experts believe that carrying extra weight may reduce blood flow to your bladder or interfere with nerve impulses there.

What's your BMI?

Height	Normal		Overweight					Obese				
BMI	19	24	25	26	27	28	29	30	35	40	45	50
Height	Weight in pounds											
4'10"	91	115	119	124	129	134	138	143	167	191	215	239
4'11"	94	119	124	128	133	138	143	148	173	198	222	247
5'0"	97	123	128	133	138	143	148	153	179	204	230	255
5'1"	100	127	132	137	143	148	153	158	185	211	238	264
5'2"	104	131	136	142	147	153	158	164	191	218	246	273
5'3"	107	135	141	146	152	158	163	169	197	225	254	282
5'4"	110	140	145	151	157	163	169	174	204	232	262	291
5'5"	114	144	150	156	162	168	174	180	210	240	270	300
5'6"	118	148	155	161	167	173	179	186	216	247	278	309
5'7"	121	153	159	166	172	178	185	191	223	255	287	319
5'8"	125	158	164	171	177	184	190	197	230	262	295	328
5'9"	128	162	169	176	182	189	196	203	236	270	304	338
5'10"	132	167	174	181	188	195	202	209	243	278	313	348
5'11"	136	172	179	186	193	200	208	215	250	286	322	358
6'0"	140	177	184	191	199	206	213	221	258	294	331	368
6'1"	144	182	189	197	204	212	219	227	265	302	340	378
6'2"	148	186	194	202	210	218	225	233	272	311	350	389
6'3"	152	192	200	208	216	224	232	240	279	319	359	399
6'4"	156	197	205	213	221	230	238	246	287	328	369	410

Source: National Institutes of Health (NIH), 1998

In general, the higher your body mass index (BMI), the more likely you are to experience urinary incontinence. If your BMI is between 25 and 29, you're considered overweight. A BMI of 30 or higher is considered obese. Research also suggests women who are obese tend to have more severe incontinence than do other women.

If you think your weight may be contributing to the problem of urinary incontinence, talk with your doctor about a safe and healthy way to shed some pounds. Losing just 5 percent to 10 percent of your body weight may significantly reduce the pressure within your abdomen that puts added stress on your bladder. In fact, studies suggest that losing weight can improve and reduce incontinence symptoms. Use the chart above to determine your BMI.

Lack of physical fitness

People who are generally fit tend also to have strong pelvic floor muscles. When you're not as fit as you should be, your pelvic floor muscles may be somewhat weak, which may contribute to urinary incontinence.

If a lack of physical fitness may increase your risk of urinary incontinence, being more physically active seems to decrease that risk. One study found that men who walked just two or three hours a week had a 25 percent lower risk of developing an enlarged prostate, compared with men who didn't exercise. Benign prostatic hyperplasia — the medical term for an enlarged prostate — can contribute to urinary incontinence. As the gland enlarges, it can constrict the urethra and block the flow of urine. For some men this problem results in urge or overflow incontinence.

Physical activity appears to be helpful for women, too. In a study of nearly 28,000 Norwegian women, researchers found that exercising at a low intensity for an hour or more each week slightly decreased the risk of urinary incontinence. Exercising for three or more hours each week had a slightly more positive effect.

There's been some speculation that vigorous physical activity may cause urinary incontinence — not protect against it. High-impact sports, such as running, basketball or gymnastics, can cause episodes of incontinence in otherwise healthy women. These vigorous activities put sudden, strong pressure on your bladder, allowing urine to leak past your urethral sphincter. However, no data links high-impact sports to an increased risk of chronic stress incontinence.

If you're having problems with incontinence and would like to become more physically active, talk with your doctor about an exercise plan that's right for you.

Persistent causes of urinary incontinence

Persistent, underlying causes of urinary incontinence include aging, menopause, previous abdominal or pelvic surgery, radiation treatment and several medical conditions. When these factors are involved, urinary incontinence may be chronic. However, treatment can improve or reduce urinary incontinence, even if the root cause of the problem persists. Here's a brief description of underlying causes of chronic urinary incontinence.

Aging

Urinary incontinence is not a given as you grow older. However, aging is a risk factor for loss of bladder control. Most studies show that the prevalence of urinary incontinence rises steadily with age.

Why is that? As you get older, many changes occur in the organs, tissues and supporting structures of your urinary system. The muscles in your bladder and urethra lose some of their strength. These age-related changes decrease your bladder's capacity to store urine, which means you have to urinate more often. If you don't heed the call promptly enough, urinary incontinence can result. Your bladder walls also become less elastic as they age — and therefore less able to contract and expel urine. In fact, studies show that, compared with younger adults, older adults tend to retain a higher volume of urine in the bladder after urination. This is known as postvoid residual volume, and it can contribute to urinary incontinence. With age, your pelvic floor muscles can also become weaker, further compromising your ability to hold urine.

Research also suggests that your bladder muscle (detrusor) becomes more active with age. An overactive bladder muscle creates the urge to urinate before your bladder is full, which can lead to urinary incontinence. In many older adults, the detrusor muscle contracts too often, but the contractions are weak. This condition — known as detrusor hyperactivity with impaired contractility (DHIC) — creates the worst of both worlds. You have frequent, sometimes uncontrollable urges to urinate, but you can't quite completely empty your bladder. This can lead to both urge incontinence and overflow incontinence.

As you age, your kidneys also become less efficient at removing waste from your bloodstream. This age-related decline in filtration can cause you to produce more urine later in the day. In fact, unlike younger people, who produce most of their urine during the day, older adults produce roughly the same amount of urine during the day and night. Having to urinate several times a night sometimes causes incontinence.

As you age, you're also more likely to have medical problems, such as congestive heart failure, diabetes or Alzheimer's disease, that can contribute to urinary incontinence. Age-related problems that restrict mobility, such as severe arthritis or hip fracture, also can lead to the problem.

In older men, incontinence often stems from enlargement of the prostate gland, a condition also known as benign prostatic hyperplasia (BPH). Around age 40, the prostate begins to enlarge slightly. As the gland enlarges, it can constrict the urethra and partially block the flow of urine. For some men, this problem results in urge or overflow incontinence. For more information on BPH and urinary incontinence, see Chapter 7.

Menopause

In women, the hormone estrogen helps keep the lining of the bladder and urethra healthy. After menopause a woman's body produces less estrogen. With less estrogen, the tissues lining the urethra become drier, thinner and less elastic. The urethral sphincter, in fact, often loses some of its ability to close — meaning that it can't hold back urine as easily as before. This can cause you to leak urine when you cough, laugh, sneeze or lift something heavy (stress incontinence). The hormonal changes of menopause can also make women more prone to urinary tract infections, which sometimes can cause urinary incontinence.

Urinary incontinence may appear for the first time after menopause, or it may worsen then. Some women have no problems with urine leakage until several years after menopause, when estrogen levels in the urethral lining fall so low that they can't support the growth of new cells.

Doctors and scientists don't yet completely understand how estrogen loss and menopause contribute to urinary incontinence. In fact, some studies comparing premenopausal and postmenopausal women have found no differences in the overall rates of urinary incontinence. Research suggests, however, that postmenopausal women tend to have more frequent problems with urine leakage

than do younger women. In one study, 7 percent of post-meno-
pausal women said they were incontinent at least once a day.
Among premenopausal women, the number was just 3 percent.

Previous surgery
In women, the bladder and uterus lie close to each other and are
supported by the same muscles and ligaments. Radical pelvic
surgery to treat cancers of the reproductive system and colon carries the risk of damaging the muscles and nerves of the urinary
tract, which can lead to urinary incontinence. Damage to the nerves
supplying the bladder may cause urine retention and overflow
incontinence, while damage to the nerves supplying the urethra or
bladder neck may cause stress incontinence.

However, studies examining the link between surgical removal
of the uterus (hysterectomy) and urinary incontinence have pro-
duced conflicting results. Some have found a strong relationship —
others have found none at all. More research is needed to clarify
the issue.

In men, the picture is clearer. Urinary incontinence is a known
side effect of prostate surgery. During radical prostatectomy for
prostate cancer, your surgeon uses special techniques to completely
remove your prostate and sometimes the surrounding lymph nodes
as well, while trying to spare the muscles and nerves that control
urination and sexual function. But sometimes the urinary sphincter
or the nerves supplying it are damaged. After the urinary catheter
is removed — typically a week or two after surgery — most men
who've undergone radical prostatectomy experience bladder control problems. These problems may last for weeks or even months.

Most men eventually regain complete bladder control, but others may leak urine when they sneeze, cough, laugh or lift something heavy. Stress incontinence is the most common type of incontinence after radical prostatectomy, but prostate surgery can also
sometimes trigger urge or overflow incontinence.

For many men who've had prostate cancer, normal bladder control gradually returns within several weeks or months of a radical
prostatectomy. But in some men, major urinary leakage persists.
Additional surgery may be needed to help correct the problem.

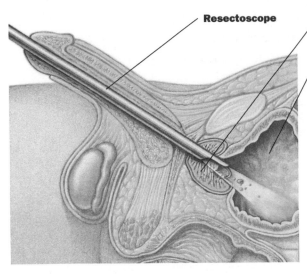

Resectoscope

Prostate gland
enlarged by BPH

Bladder

Transurethral resection of the
prostate (TURP) is the most
common surgery for benign
prostatic hyperplasia (BPH).
A thin instrument (resectoscope) is threaded through
the urethra to where it's surrounded by the prostate. Tiny
cutting tools on the resectoscope scrape away excess
prostate tissue, improving
urine flow.

Other prostate surgeries also may cause urinary incontinence.
For example, transurethral resection of the prostate (TURP), the
most common surgery for an enlarged prostate, usually relieves
urinary symptoms. Most men experience a stronger urine flow
within a few days after surgery. But in some cases TURP can cause
loss of bladder control. This condition is usually temporary, but it
can take up to a year for it to disappear entirely. Complete removal
of the prostate gland (open prostatectomy) is a more invasive
surgery generally reserved for excessively enlarged prostates. It's a
safe and effective therapy, although the procedure does pose the
risk of side effects, including urinary incontinence. In addition, its
side effects tend to be more pronounced.

For more information on urinary incontinence and prostate
surgery, see Chapter 7. This chapter also contains additional information on the possible link between hysterectomy and urinary
incontinence.

Radiation treatment

Normally, your bladder stretches as it fills with urine. The fuller it
gets, the more it stretches. Pelvic radiation therapy can damage
your bladder wall, making it somewhat stiff. This loss of elasticity
can cause increased urinary frequency and urgency and sometimes
results in urinary incontinence.

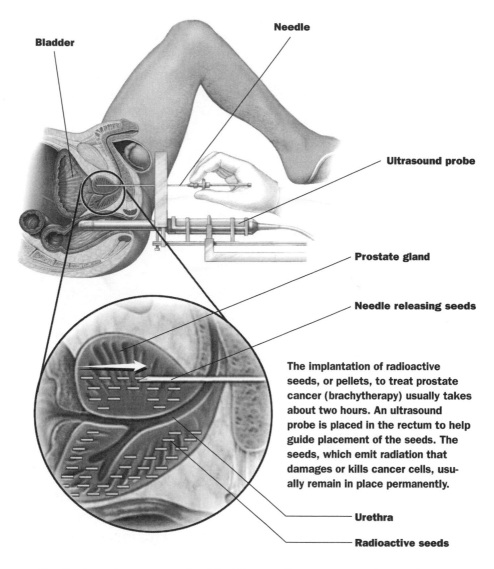

Bladder

Needle

Ultrasound probe

Prostate gland

Needle releasing seeds

The implantation of radioactive seeds, or pellets, to treat prostate cancer (brachytherapy) usually takes about two hours. An ultrasound probe is placed in the rectum to help guide placement of the seeds. The seeds, which emit radiation that damages or kills cancer cells, usually remain in place permanently.

Urethra

Radioactive seeds

Radiation damage to the bladder wall can occur after radiation therapy for gynecologic, urologic or colorectal cancers. During external beam radiation treatment for prostate cancer, the most common urinary problems are increased urgency and frequency. These problems usually are temporary and gradually diminish within a few weeks of completing treatment. Long-term problems are uncommon. According to the American Cancer Society, fewer than 5 percent of men treated with external beam radiation therapy use absorbent pads for urinary incontinence.

With radioactive seed implants (brachytherapy), it's a slightly different story. Seed implants deliver a higher dose of radiation to the urethra, causing urinary problems in nearly all men. Some men need medication to treat these signs and symptoms. Some may also need medications or intermittent self-catheterization to help them urinate.

In general, urinary problems tend to be more pronounced and longer lasting with seed implants than with external beam radiation. Severe urinary incontinence isn't a common side effect of seed implants. However, the American Cancer Society reports that increased urinary frequency persists in about one-third of men who've undergone brachytherapy for prostate cancer.

Congestive heart failure

Congestive heart failure often occurs because other cardiovascular diseases have damaged or weakened your heart, forcing it to work harder. It can result from a heart attack, high blood pressure or other forms of heart disease, such as valve disorders. Because your heart is weakened, it can't pump blood efficiently. This causes blood to pool in your legs, feet and ankles, causing swelling. The medical term for this condition is peripheral edema. Your kidneys also retain excess water and sodium, and fluid backs up into your lungs, leading to shortness of breath.

When fluid builds up in your body due to congestive heart failure, the fluid can cause or contribute to incontinence. With excess fluid in your body, you have to urinate more frequently. If you're not strong enough to get to the bathroom quickly, urinary incontinence can result. Congestive heart failure and peripheral edema also appear to lead to increased production of urine at night, which can contribute to urinary incontinence. Sometimes, the simple act of lying flat is enough to cause urine leakage. When you lie down, excess fluid moves from your lower extremities, sometimes creating pressure on your bladder and an uncontrollable urge to urinate.

Diuretics are a mainstay of treatment for congestive heart failure. They make you urinate more frequently and keep fluid from collecting in your body. But they, too, can contribute to urinary incontinence.

Diabetes

When you have diabetes, your body processes blood sugar (glucose) in an abnormal way. Instead of being transported into your cells, glucose accumulates in your bloodstream and is eventually excreted in your urine. This usually occurs either because your body doesn't produce enough insulin or because your body doesn't respond to insulin properly.

As a disease, diabetes can cause or contribute to urinary incontinence in several different ways. Excess glucose circulating in your body draws water from your tissues, making you feel dehydrated. To quench your thirst, you may drink a lot of water and other beverages, leading to more frequent urination and sometimes to urinary incontinence. In fact, uncontrolled diabetes with associated high blood sugar (hyperglycemia) is one of the most common causes of excess urine production.

Diabetes also increases your risk of developing urinary tract infections. These infections irritate the bladder, causing strong urges to urinate. When the urge is so strong that you can't get to the toilet in time, urinary incontinence can result.

Nerve damage (neuropathy) is another complication of diabetes that can lead to urinary incontinence. Damage to the nerves that control urination can cause faulty communication between your brain and your urinary tract. This can cause a reduced sensation to urinate, even when your bladder is full, which can cause overflow incontinence. Nerve damage from diabetes also may prevent your bladder from emptying completely (urinary retention), contributing to overflow incontinence and urinary tract infections. If urinary retention isn't properly treated, urine can back up into your kidneys. Called vesicoureteral reflux, this can result in damage to kidney function.

Diabetes also can affect your kidneys more generally, damaging the intricate system that filters waste from your blood and eliminates it in your urine. Over time, kidney damage from diabetes (nephropathy) can cause chronic kidney failure. That, in turn, can cause fluid retention, leading to swollen extremities, congestive heart failure or fluid in your lungs. Urinary incontinence can be another consequence of retaining excess fluid.

Neurological disorders

Disorders of your brain and spinal cord can affect bladder control by interrupting the nerve impulses that normally get sent to your bladder. Neurological disorders that can cause urinary incontinence include multiple sclerosis, Parkinson's disease, stroke, Alzheimer's disease, spinal cord injury, spinal stenosis, and normal pressure hydrocephalus, among others. Often, these disorders cause your bladder muscle to become overactive. When the bladder muscle is overactive because of a neurological disease or disorder, the condition is known as neurologic hyperreflexia.

The mechanism behind urinary incontinence is slightly different for each neurological disorder. Here's a brief summary:

Multiple sclerosis. In multiple sclerosis, your immune system mistakenly attacks the myelin sheath surrounding the nerves in your brain and spinal cord. The resulting injury and scarring slows or blocks muscle coordination and other nerve signals, often causing bladder overactivity, urinary frequency and sometimes incontinence. Nerve damage from multiple sclerosis can also make your bladder muscle underactive, contributing to overflow incontinence. Doctors estimate that about 80 percent of people with multiple sclerosis have urinary problems.

Parkinson's disease. Parkinson's disease occurs when neurons in the area of your brain that controls muscle movement are damaged or destroyed. This can cause both uncontrollable muscle movements (tremors) and muscle stiffness (rigidity). If you have Parkinson's, your bladder muscle may become overactive, contributing to urge incontinence, or underactive, contributing to overflow incontinence. The slowed movement and muscle stiffness associated with Parkinson's disease can also make it difficult to get to the toilet in time.

Stroke. A stroke can contribute to urinary incontinence in several different ways. If the bladder control center of the brain is damaged by the stroke itself or the subsequent swelling, you may be unable to sense or suppress the urge to urinate. Control of your bladder muscle also may be impaired, causing hyperreflexia and urge incontinence. Depending on its severity, a stroke can also impair your ability to think and speak. These impairments may make you unable to recognize the urge to urinate or communicate that need to a caregiver in a timely way. Urinary incontinence is fairly common after a stroke. However, for many people, the problem improves with time and rehabilitation.

Alzheimer's disease. In Alzheimer's disease, healthy brain tissue degenerates, ultimately causing a loss of memory severe enough to interfere with daily functioning (dementia). Urinary incontinence becomes more common as the disease progresses, when thinking becomes increasingly impaired. When people with Alzheimer's disease begin to have wetting accidents, it may be because they have forgotten where the bathroom is located or they have trouble getting to it in time. Unlike other neurological disorders, Alzheimer's doesn't appear to cause unstable bladder contractions.

Spinal cord injury. An injury to the spinal cord interferes with your brain's ability to communicate through your nervous system with other parts of your body. It can stem from a sudden, traumatic blow to your spine that fractures, dislocates, crushes or compresses one or more of your vertebrae or from a penetrating wound that cuts your spinal cord. If you have paralysis from a spinal cord injury that affects the nerves running to the bladder, you may experience reflux incontinence. Damage to these nerves prevents the transfer of messages between the brain and the bladder, leading to urine loss without any sensation or warning.

Spinal stenosis. In spinal stenosis, one or more areas of the spine narrow — especially in the upper or lower back — putting pressure on the spinal cord or on the roots of its branching nerves. Most often, spinal stenosis results from degenerative changes in the spine caused by aging. But tumors, injuries and other diseases can also lead to narrowing in the spinal canal. In severe cases of spinal stenosis, nerves to the bladder may be affected, leading to partial or complete urinary incontinence. The medical term for this problem is cauda equina syndrome.

Cervical spondylosis is the medical term for degenerative changes in the bones (vertebrae) and cartilage of the neck. As the condition progresses, it can cause spinal stenosis and bladder overactivity in older adults.

Normal pressure hydrocephalus. Normal pressure hydrocephalus (NPH) is characterized by the swelling of a portion of the brain called the cerebral ventricles. The swelling is caused by an accumulation of an excessive amount of cerebrospinal fluid within the skull. With NPH, this fluid may be at the upper end of normal pressure. The swelling can damage brain tissue, leading to a number of signs and symptoms, including dementia, difficulty standing and walking, and urinary incontinence.

NPH most often occurs in people age 55 years and older. Bladder problems may range from urinary frequency and urgency in mild cases to complete loss of bladder control in advanced cases.

The next step

Urinary incontinence has a variety of causes. Some are temporary, such as drinking too many caffeinated beverages or the effects of certain medications, and can be remedied by a change in behavior. Other causes are persistent, such as the effects of aging or menopause, and the incontinence from these causes may be harder to completely overcome. Regardless of the underlying cause of urinary incontinence, there is almost always a treatment that works to at least relieve some of the signs and symptoms. In the chapters ahead, you'll find out about many treatment options that are available.

Chapter 3

Getting help

You may feel uncomfortable discussing urinary incontinence with your doctor. You're not alone — many people do. But seeking medical advice is important for several reasons. First, urinary incontinence may indicate a more serious underlying condition. Second, it may cause you to restrict your activities and limit your social interactions. Third, if you have balance problems, it may put you at risk of falling if you're rushing to the bathroom to avoid leaking urine.

A few isolated incidents of urinary incontinence don't necessarily require medical attention. But if the problem is frequent or affects your quality of life, it's important to see your doctor.

Finding a care provider

If you're having trouble with urinary incontinence, making an appointment with your primary care provider is probably a good place to start. General practitioners, family practitioners, general internists, physician assistants and nurse practitioners often can treat urinary incontinence without bringing in specialists. However, some primary care physicians don't have the necessary interest, training or experience to treat urinary incontinence. Some may take the view that urinary incontinence is an inevitable consequence of childbearing, menopause or just growing older — and that it's a waste of time to try to do anything about it.

If your primary care doctor doesn't seem to have a positive attitude about treating urinary incontinence or seems uninformed when discussing the subject, consider looking for another care provider. Another general practitioner, family practitioner or general internist may be able to provide the care and support you need.

Seeing a specialist is another possibility. There are a few different options. A urologist is a medical doctor who specializes in the male reproductive organs and the urinary disorders in both men and women. A urogynecologist is an obstetrician-gynecologist with additional training in problems affecting a woman's pelvic floor — the network of muscles, ligaments, connective tissue and nerves that help support and control the rectum, uterus, vagina and bladder. A geriatrician is a medical doctor who specializes in the care of older adults, often with special emphasis on problems related to medications and changes in bladder habits.

Your health insurance plan may require that you see a primary care doctor before getting a referral to a specialist. Other plans might let you choose a specialist without first seeing a primary care doctor.

Whether you opt for a primary care physician or a specialist, the important thing is to find a care provider who meets your needs. You can get recommendations from friends, family, a hospital you trust or your local or state medical society. Before making a decision, consider all the facts. Do you think the doctor will listen to your concerns about urinary incontinence, answer your questions and explain things clearly? Above all, ask yourself one key question: Does the doctor seem interested in treating urinary incontinence? If the answer is yes, make an appointment. With that, you'll have taken an important first step toward regaining a more active and confident life.

Preparing for a visit

To get the most from your visit to your doctor, it's important that you prepare well. Good preparation before a doctor visit for urinary incontinence generally consists of two parts. First, gather and document the facts of your medical history. This step may include getting a copy of your medical record or having it sent to the doctor you'll be seeing. Second, you need to keep a brief bladder diary. By providing this important background information, you'll give your care provider the best chance at treating your incontinence successfully. In addition, before your appointment your doctor may ask you to complete a questionnaire about your bladder function.

Recording your medical history

Before your visit to your doctor, review your medical history and make a few lists. Medications are one of the most common causes of urinary incontinence, so list all the medications you're taking. Include prescriptions, over-the-counter drugs, vitamins, minerals and other supplements. If you're not sure whether something counts as a medication, err on the side of caution and put it on the list anyway.

For each medication, write down the brand and generic names, the dose you take, how often you take it and when you take it. If you're allergic to any medications, note them. It may also be a good idea to bring your medications to your appointment. If you plan to do this, be sure to keep them in their original containers.

The time before your visit to your doctor is also a good opportunity to make some notes about your medical history. List any and all previous surgeries, births, illnesses, injuries and medical procedures, and provide approximate dates. If you have health problems for which you're currently seeing a doctor or taking medication, such as arthritis or diabetes, list those, too. For women who have been through menopause, it's also helpful to note when menstrual periods stopped. You can note the date or simply jot down how old you were when you stopped menstruating. Urinary incontinence can be the result of a urinary tract infection, so it's also a good idea to document any past or current problems with your urinary system.

Finally, if you want a report of your consultation sent to other health care providers, be sure to bring along their current addresses to the appointment.

Keeping a bladder diary

Before or after your appointment, your doctor may ask you to keep a bladder diary at home over several days. This simple record of "fluids in and fluids out" will provide important details about your incontinence symptoms. If you keep it faithfully, it will show when you're leaking urine, how often you're leaking, how much you're leaking and which situations in your life seem to be associated with episodes of urinary incontinence. With this information, your doctor will have a better idea of what might be contributing to your incontinence — and how best to treat it. See pages 188-189 of the Appendix for a sample bladder diary.

Being evaluated for urinary incontinence

Usually the next step in being evaluated for urinary incontinence is to see your doctor for a complete medical exam. The sequence and number of steps in the exam may vary, but it's likely that your doctor will ask you a series of specific questions about your signs and symptoms, followed by even more questions about your medical history. Typically, you'll also have a complete physical examination and undergo some basic tests of your urinary function. Your doctor's goal is to correlate your signs and symptoms, medical history, physical exam and test results to provide an accurate assessment of your problem.

At the end of the appointment, your doctor may prescribe a course of treatment for your urinary incontinence. However, if your tests or physical exam raises additional questions or concerns, you may need to undergo further testing.

Assessing your symptoms

Your doctor will usually begin the appointment by asking you about your signs and symptoms and medical history. How often do you need to urinate? When do you leak urine? Do you have trouble emptying your bladder? Are you experiencing any symptoms in addition to incontinence? Your answers to these questions can help your doctor determine what type of incontinence you have and how best to treat it. If you're unsure about any of your responses, your bladder diary may serve as a helpful resource.

Your doctor may first ask about the onset and duration of the problem. When did the incontinence start? Did it come on suddenly or more gradually over time? How long has it been going on? Has it gotten any better or worse? Next, there may be questions designed to uncover details about your specific problem. Here is a list of questions you might expect:

- How often do you leak urine during the day? Are you aware that it's happening or do you just find yourself wet?
- What time of day does it typically occur? Is it worse during the day or at night?
- When you leak urine, is it just a few drops? Or are your underwear or clothes soaked?
- Do you often feel a sudden and intense urge to urinate that's difficult to control?
- Do you feel the urge to urinate when you hear the sound of running water?
- Do you feel the urge to urinate when you put your hands in warm water?
- Do you leak urine when you laugh, cough, sneeze or lift heavy objects?
- Do you leak urine when you exercise?
- How often do you urinate in the toilet during the day? Do you urinate more than eight times in a 24-hour period? Do you urinate frequently, but only a small amount each time?
- Do you wake at least twice during the night to urinate?
- Do you ever wake up wet?
- Do you feel pain, discomfort, or a burning or smarting sensation while urinating?
- Have you ever seen blood in your urine?
- Does your urine ever look cloudy?
- Do you have trouble starting the urine stream?
- Do you have a slow or weak urine stream?
- Does your urine stream start and stop?
- Does your bladder sometimes feel full even after you urinate?
- Do you have to bear down or strain to urinate?

- Do you dribble urine after you're done urinating?
- What's your typical daily fluid intake?
- Do you tend to drink more in the morning, afternoon or evening?
- Do you drink caffeinated beverages? How many each day?
- Do you drink alcoholic beverages? How many each day?
- Have you noticed any recent changes in your bowel habits?
- How often do you have bowel movements?
- Are you often constipated?
- Have you had any problems with fecal incontinence?
- Have you noticed any recent changes in your sexual function?
- Do you leak urine during or after sexual intercourse?
- Are you still having menstrual periods (women only)?
- Do you use absorbent pads to protect your clothes from wetting accidents?
- How many pads do you use a day? What type?
- Are the pads usually soaked or just damp?
- Does anything seem to make your urinary incontinence better or worse? If so, what?
- What's the most bothersome aspect of your problem with urinary incontinence?

After getting a good sense of your urinary symptoms, your doctor may move on to aspects of your medical history that may be causing or contributing to urinary incontinence. The medical history information you've gathered to prepare for the appointment can help you answer most of these questions. Current or past medical problems that can affect bladder control include urinary tract infection, prostate enlargement, diabetes, stroke, Parkinson's disease and multiple sclerosis, among others. For women, menopause also can contribute to urinary incontinence. For more information on the different medical conditions that can cause or contribute to urinary incontinence, see Chapter 2.

Next, you may be asked about any previous surgeries or radiation therapy. Gynecologic and urologic procedures, such as hysterectomy, radical prostatectomy or radioactive seed implants for prostate cancer (brachytherapy), have perhaps the strongest association with urinary incontinence. But it's important to mention any procedures you've had — including any prior surgeries to treat urinary incontinence. Any surgery in which you were catheterized with a Foley catheter may have caused scarring of your urethral lining, which may now be contributing to urinary incontinence.

If you've been pregnant or given birth, your doctor may have some questions about that, too. How many times have you been pregnant? How many times have you given birth? What was the size of each baby? Did you deliver vaginally or by Caesarean section? Did you have an episiotomy? Were forceps used? Was the birth assisted with a vacuum device? With this information, your doctor will begin to get an idea about the general condition of your pelvic floor.

Your doctor may also ask you about the medications you're currently taking, including prescriptions, over-the-counter drugs, vitamins, minerals and other supplements. Again, the information you've gathered to prepare for the appointment should help you answer these questions. Because medications are such a common cause of urinary incontinence, it's important to discuss the subject thoroughly. After reviewing your specific circumstances, your doctor may recommend that some of your medications be reduced, discontinued or taken at different times of the day.

Quality of life assessment

Urinary incontinence can cause many unpleasant side effects, such as rashes, skin infections and sores from constantly wet skin. But more distressing than these physical problems may be the effect urinary incontinence can have on your quality of life.

Urinary incontinence may keep you from participating in activities. You may stop exercising, quit attending social gatherings or even refrain from laughing because you're afraid of an accident. You may even reach the point where you stop traveling or venturing out of familiar areas where you know the locations of toilets.

Urinary incontinence may also negatively affect your work life. Your urge to urinate may keep you away from your desk or cause you to have to get up often during meetings. The problem may be so distressing that it disrupts your concentration. Urinary incontinence may also keep you up at night, so you're tired most of the time.

Perhaps most distressing is the effect urinary incontinence can have on your personal life. Your family may not understand the changes in your behavior or may grow frustrated at your many trips to the bathroom. You may avoid sexual intimacy because of embarrassment caused by urine leakage. It's not uncommon to experience anxiety and depression along with urinary incontinence.

To fully understand how urinary incontinence is affecting your quality of life, your doctor may ask you to complete a questionnaire, such as the Incontinence Impact Questionnaire (IIQ), the Urogenital Distress Inventory (UDI) or the International Prostate Symptom Score (IPSS — for men only). The questionnaires ask you to rate how urine leakage has affected the different aspects of your life, such as physical recreation, travel, sexual relations and participation in social activities outside your home. They also ask you to describe how leaking urine makes you feel, whether it be nervous, fearful, frustrated, angry, depressed or embarrassed.

With the results of the questionnaire, your doctor can get a clearer picture of how urinary incontinence is affecting your everyday life. This information may help your doctor devise treatment strategies to address the areas that are most troublesome to you.

Physical examination

A complete physical examination, with extra focus on your abdomen, genital area, rectum and nervous system, can provide important clues to the cause of your incontinence.

Your doctor may begin the exam by assessing your general mobility and dexterity. You may be asked to show how you pull your clothes up and down and fasten and unfasten buttons, belts and zippers in order to urinate. Or your doctor may simply observe how easily you can climb onto the exam table. If you're having trouble moving or undressing, that may be contributing to your incontinence.

Your doctor will also likely check your vital signs and check for swelling (edema) in your legs, ankles and feet. Lower extremity edema, often a consequence of congestive heart failure, diabetes or kidney failure, contributes to increased urine production at night, which sometimes leads to urinary incontinence.

If your bladder is full, your doctor may perform a test for stress incontinence. The test is slightly different for men and women. Men are asked to stand up and cough. If urine leaks out onto a paper towel, the test is positive for stress incontinence. Women are asked to cough while lying on the exam table. If no urine leaks out, they're asked to stand up and cough again, bounce on their heels, walk or bend over. You shouldn't be embarrassed if you leak urine during a stress test. Think of it as an important part of beginning to understand your problem. Once the test is over, you can urinate so that you're comfortable for the rest of the exam. Your doctor may observe you as you urinate to see whether your urine flow is strong and continuous. If your urine flow is weak, intermittent or if you're straining to urinate, you may have overflow incontinence.

Once your bladder is empty, your doctor may perform an abdominal exam by pushing on your abdomen and listening for bowel sounds. If your bladder seems to be larger than it should be (bladder distention), it may mean that it's not emptying completely when you urinate, which could be contributing to overflow incontinence. Soreness or tenderness in the area over your bladder is another symptom of bladder distention. If your doctor doesn't hear bowel sounds, you may be constipated, which could be contributing to your incontinence. The abdominal exam will also allow your doctor to check for other abdominal factors that may be contributing to incontinence, such as a hernia, tumor, infection or scarring from previous surgery.

Your doctor may also perform a brief neurological exam, testing your reflexes with a reflex hammer and assessing the strength of your leg muscles. In addition, your doctor may check to see whether you can feel it when your legs are being touched with a pin — and whether you can distinguish the sharp pin from a duller instrument. During this part of the physical exam, your doctor is trying to determine whether neurological disorders such as multiple sclerosis, Parkinson's disease or spinal stenosis may be interrupting or weakening the nerve impulses that normally get sent to your bladder — and therefore contributing to your incontinence.

Pelvic and rectal exams for women

For women, the physical exam also focuses on the reproductive organs and rectum. During a pelvic exam, you lie on your back on an examining table with your knees bent. Usually, your heels rest in metal supports called stirrups.

Your doctor will likely examine your external genitalia (vulva) and the area between your vulva and anus, called the perineum. Chronic exposure to urine can cause skin problems on your perineum and external genitals, such as rashes, sores and infection. To test the nerves in your genital area, your doctor may lightly scratch the perineal skin near your anus and watch or feel for an anal contraction. This reflex is sometimes known as the anal wink. Your doctor may also lightly squeeze your clitoris and look for a similar anal contraction. This reflex is known as the bulbocavernosus reflex. If these reflexes aren't normal, it may mean that the nerves in your genital area are somehow contributing to your problem with urinary incontinence. These tests may feel a bit unusual, but they shouldn't be painful.

The internal examination is usually next. It allows your doctor to evaluate the condition of your vagina, assess the strength of your pelvic floor muscles, determine whether your bladder or uterus has dropped out of its normal position (pelvic organ prolapse) and detect any abnormal masses. Vaginal atrophy, weak pelvic floor muscles, pelvic organ prolapse and abnormal pelvic masses can all contribute to urinary incontinence.

To begin the internal exam, your doctor inserts an instrument called a speculum into your vagina. With the speculum in the open position, your doctor checks for inflammation or discharge, which may suggest a vaginal infection. He or she may also be able to see whether your vaginal walls are thinning. Often, if your vaginal walls are thinning, the tissues lining your urethra are thinning, too, which may contribute to urinary incontinence.

After examining your vagina, your doctor may insert one or two gloved fingers into your vagina to help assess the strength of your pelvic floor muscles and determine whether your bladder and uterus are in the proper position. Some doctors use the speculum to do this exam. You'll likely be asked to cough or squeeze your pelvic muscles as if you're trying to stop your urine stream. If your doctor suspects that you have a pelvic organ prolapse, you may be asked to repeat this test while sitting or standing. In these positions, the prolapse may become more pronounced. To complete your internal exam, your doctor may check your uterus and ovaries for any abnormal masses. This is done by inserting two gloved fingers into your vagina and pressing down on your abdomen with the other hand.

Another step is the digital rectal exam. To do this, your doctor inserts a gloved finger into your rectum to check for any masses or impacted stool, which may be contributing to urinary incontinence. A rectal exam can also help your doctor judge the strength of your pelvic floor muscles. To help determine the strength of these muscles, your doctor may ask you to squeeze your anus around the examining finger, as if you're trying to avoid urinating or passing gas.

Genital, rectal and prostate exams for men

For men, the physical exam next focuses on the penis, perineum, testicles, rectum and prostate gland. Your doctor may first examine your penis and the area between your scrotum and anus, called the

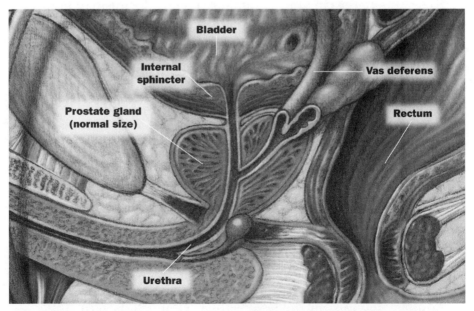

This cross-sectional view shows the prostate gland (center) and surrounding structures. When it becomes enlarged, the prostate can interfere with the flow of urine through the urethra.

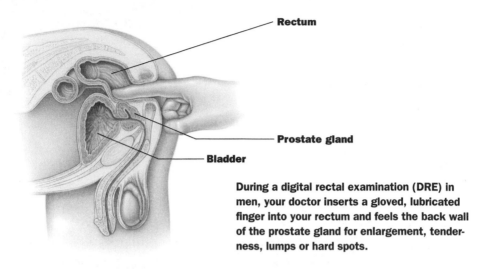

Rectum

Prostate gland

Bladder

During a digital rectal examination (DRE) in men, your doctor inserts a gloved, lubricated finger into your rectum and feels the back wall of the prostate gland for enlargement, tenderness, lumps or hard spots.

perineum. Chronic exposure to urine can cause skin problems on the foreskin, the head of the penis (glans penis) and the perineum. Sometimes this leads to swelling or enlargement of the penis. If you have not been circumcised, your doctor will pull the foreskin back to inspect the glans. Your doctor may also check for abnormal narrowing of your urethra, which can be caused by scarring or infection.

To test the nerves in your genital area, your doctor may lightly scratch the perineal skin near your anus and watch or feel for an anal contraction. This reflex is sometimes called the anal wink. Your doctor may also lightly squeeze the glans penis and look for a similar anal contraction. This reflex is known as the bulbocavernosus reflex. If these reflexes aren't normal, it may mean that the nerves in your genital area are somehow contributing to your problem with urinary incontinence. These tests may feel a bit unusual, but they shouldn't be painful.

Another part of the exam may include your testicles. Each testicle may be checked for symmetry, inflammation and unusual growths. The coiled tube at the top and rear of each testicle, called the epididymis, may be checked for scarring. Scarring of the epididymis, which is a sign of previous infections, often accompanies prostate infection (prostatitis) and its associated urinary problems.

Another step in your physical is the digital rectal exam. Your doctor inserts a gloved finger into your rectum to check the size, symmetry and texture of your prostate gland. If your prostate is enlarged or infected, it may be preventing your bladder from emptying completely, which may be causing your incontinence. The digital rectal exam also allows your doctor to check for any masses or impacted stool, which can contribute to urinary incontinence. Plus, it can help demonstrate the strength of your pelvic floor muscles. To help determine the strength of these muscles, your doctor may ask you to squeeze your anus around the examining finger, as if you're trying to avoid urinating or passing gas.

Urinalysis

Urinalysis is a routine part of being evaluated for urinary incontinence. A sample of your urine is sent to a laboratory, where it's checked for blood, glucose, bacteria or other abnormalities. For the sample to be collected, you're asked to urinate into a container.

Blood in your urine may indicate an irritation of your urinary tract, such as an infection, urinary stone or tumor. If you have blood in your urine, your doctor may prescribe another test to rule out the possibility of bladder cancer. This test, called urine cytology, specifically checks the urine for cancer cells.

If glucose is detected in your urine, your doctor may suspect diabetes, which can increase your urine volume and make incontinence more likely. More testing can help confirm the diagnosis.

Bacteria in your urine can be a sign of urinary tract infection. To get more information about the specific microbe causing the infection, your doctor may send your urine to a laboratory to be cultured. This is called a urine culture test. If the culture is positive, you'll likely be prescribed a course of antibiotics.

Postvoid residual test

This test, known as PVR, helps your doctor determine whether you have difficulty emptying your bladder. It measures the amount of urine left in your bladder in the five to 10 minutes after you urinate. A bladder that doesn't empty completely can lead to increased urinary frequency and can make stress incontinence worse.

For the procedure, you urinate (void) into a container that allows your doctor to measure your urine output. Your doctor then quickly checks the amount of residual urine in your bladder in one of two ways. One option is to insert a thin, soft tube (catheter) into your urethra and bladder to drain any remaining urine. This provides a clean sample for urine culture and prepares you for additional tests, but it's invasive and can be a bit uncomfortable. It also poses a small risk of urinary tract infection.

The other option, which is painless, is to gauge the amount of residual urine using an ultrasound device. For the ultrasound test, a wand-like device that sends sound waves is placed over your abdomen and pelvic area. A computer transforms these sound waves into an image of your bladder, so your doctor can see how full or empty it is. This option is quicker and less painful than catheterization. Plus, the ultrasound images can provide your doctor with important information about the overall condition and capacity of your bladder.

Some amount of residual urine is normal. A normal PVR reading may be as high as 60 milliliters (2 ounces), even higher among older people. A reading over 250 milliliters or 25 percent of your total bladder capacity is generally considered abnormal. If your PVR reading is in this range after repeated tests, it may mean that you have an obstruction in your urinary tract or a problem with your bladder nerves or muscles.

Beginning conservative therapy

After reviewing your symptoms, medical history, physical exam and test results, your doctor may prescribe a course of treatment for your urinary incontinence. The first step is to try what are called conservative therapies. These treatments don't involve surgery. They include behavioral techniques such as bladder training, scheduled toilet trips, pelvic floor muscle (Kegel) exercises and fluid and diet management.

Medications are another form of conservative therapy for urinary incontinence. Drugs commonly used to treat urinary incontinence include tolterodine (Detrol), oxybutynin (Ditropan), hyoscyamine (Levsin) and trospium (Sanctura). The antidepressant imipramine (Tofranil) also may be used to treat urinary incontinence. In addition, a drug called duloxetine (Cymbalta), currently used to treat peripheral neuropathy and depression, is being evaluated for use in treating urinary incontinence.

When other tests may be needed

If conservative therapies aren't successful, or your problem isn't easily diagnosed by basic urinary tests, a thorough physical exam and a discussion of your symptoms, your doctor may recommend further evaluation. If you haven't been seeing a specialist, you may be referred to a urologist or urogynecologist.

The specialist may repeat the basic evaluation done previously plus do additional tests. Such tests might include the following.

Cystoscopy

This procedure allows your doctor to see the inside of your urethra and bladder. A thin tube with a tiny lens (cystoscope) is inserted into your urethra and bladder, and your bladder is filled with sterile fluid. Stretching your bladder with fluid gives your doctor a better view of your bladder wall. Your doctor then checks your bladder and urethra for potential causes of urinary incontinence. Bladder infections, tumors, abscesses, stones and other abnormalities can cause urinary incontinence. Other contributing factors can include problems with your urethra, such as pouches or sac openings (urethral diverticula) or urethral narrowing caused by scar tissue, or an obstructing prostate gland (urethral stricture). During the procedure, your doctor may use the cystoscope to remove a small sample of bladder tissue for lab analysis or even to remove a small stone.

Cystoscopy typically takes about 15 to 20 minutes from start to finish, including preparation time. You usually are given a local anesthetic in gel form (no injection) and remain awake during the brief procedure. You may feel some discomfort and the need to urinate as your bladder fills. After the test, your urethra may be sore and you may have a mild burning feeling when you urinate. You may also see small amounts of blood in your urine. These problems

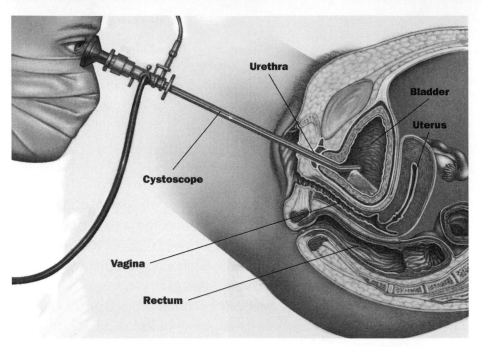

Labels in image:
Urethra
Bladder
Uterus
Cystoscope
Vagina
Rectum

Cystoscopic examination allows your doctor to see inside your urethra and bladder. It can help in diagnosing urethral and bladder problems that cause urinary incontinence.

usually go away within a few days. If problems persist or you develop signs or symptoms of infection, including a burning sensation when you urinate, cloudy urine, fever or chills, call your doctor.

Intravenous pyelogram

An intravenous pyelogram (IVP) — sometimes called an excretory urogram — is an X-ray examination used to gauge kidney function and the drainage of urine through the urinary tract. It provides your doctor with a detailed view of your kidneys, ureters and bladder and often is used to identify potential reasons for blood in your urine.

During an IVP test, you receive an injection of dye through a vein in your arm. Your bloodstream rapidly delivers the dye to your kidneys, where it passes through the intricate filtration system. Later, the dye flows down your ureters and into your bladder. As the dye outlines the organs and structures of your urinary tract, a series of X-rays is taken. These X-rays show any tumors, cysts, stones, scarring and areas where fluid may be building up or escaping.

An IVP typically takes about an hour. You will probably have no side effects, although some people report nausea, vomiting or pain at the injection site. If you're allergic to seafood, iodine or radiologic contrast agents, tell your doctor before having an IVP. Allergic reactions to the contrast dye sometimes do occur. If you're pregnant, you should not have an IVP test unless it's an emergency. The radiation may harm your baby.

Urodynamic study

Urodynamic study (UDS) is the general term for tests that show the urinary system in action. Urodynamic testing will likely be recommended if your symptoms seem to indicate mixed incontinence, if you've had previous surgery on your bladder or sphincter, or if conservative therapies for incontinence aren't working. It's also most always recommended before surgery for incontinence.

There are several different urodynamic tests that make up a urodynamic study. They include the following:

Uroflowmetry. This test measures how fast your urine comes out, in milliliters per second. You start with a full bladder and urinate into a funnel at a special commode that automatically calculates your rate of flow. You'll likely be given some privacy to do this. If your peak or average flow rate is lower than normal, you may have an obstruction in your urethra or a weak bladder muscle.

Cystometry. This test measures the volume and pressure in your bladder — when it's at rest, as it fills with urine and as you urinate.

After your bladder is completely empty, a catheter is inserted into your urethra and bladder to measure the pressure. A small pressure monitor also may be inserted into the vagina (for women) or rectum. The separate catheter is then used to fill your bladder with warm, sterile water. As your bladder fills, the pressure within your bladder is recorded. Normally, pressure increases by only very small amounts during filling. However, in some people with urinary incontinence,

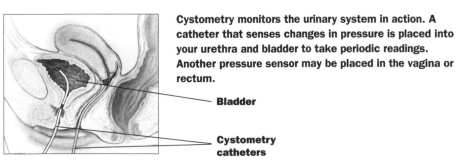

Cystometry monitors the urinary system in action. A catheter that senses changes in pressure is placed into your urethra and bladder to take periodic readings. Another pressure sensor may be placed in the vagina or rectum.

Bladder

Cystometry catheters

the bladder goes into spasms as it fills. This test also helps your doctor measure the strength of your bladder muscle.

During the test, you'll be asked when you first feel the urge to urinate and when that urge becomes strong. You'll also be asked to cough or bear down at several points. The bladder pressure at which you leak urine when you cough or strain is called the abdominal leak point pressure. At the end of the test, you urinate into the special commode, with the pressure sensors still in place. You'll have privacy to do this. This is also known as a voiding pressure test. Last, the pressure-sensing catheter will be slowly drawn through your urethra to measure the urethra's ability to close. This part of the test is called the urethral pressure profile.

After the test, you may have increased urinary frequency and urgency. Your urine may be slightly pink for about a day. If these problems persist or you develop signs of infection, call your doctor.

Electromyography. This test, also known as EMG, measures muscle activity and helps determine whether the bladder and urethra are working together properly. Small adhesive electrode patches, similar to those used during an electrocardiogram test, are placed on the skin near your urethra and rectum. A machine then records the electrical current created when your pelvic floor muscles contract. EMG is typically recommended when your doctor suspects that your incontinence is related to nerve damage.

Cystography. In this special X-ray of the bladder, also known as a cystogram or voiding cystourethrogram (VCUG), a catheter is inserted into your urethra and bladder. Through the catheter, your doctor injects a fluid containing a special dye. As this dye moves through your urinary tract and out of your body through urination, a series of X-ray images is taken. These images can help reveal problems with your urinary tract.

A cystogram may be done in conjunction with uroflowmetry or cystometry, or both. The test — called a video urodynamics study — takes about an hour. After the test, you may have some pain while urinating and your urine might be slightly pink. If these problems persist or you develop signs of infection, call your doctor.

Once all your tests are complete, your doctor can explain the results and discuss treatment options with you.

Chapter 4

Behavior therapies for urinary incontinence

There are a variety of treatments for urinary incontinence. Which one is best depends on the type of incontinence you have, whether you're a woman or a man, and how much incontinence affects your daily life. Most doctors start out with conservative treatment that's minimally invasive or noninvasive and has proven benefits, little risk and few side effects. If this doesn't work, you and your doctor may consider additional care, including more-invasive procedures. These treatments may have more side effects, but offer greater relief.

This chapter deals with behavior therapies — changes you can make to improve urinary incontinence. These changes are safe, easy, effective and inexpensive. For this reason, your doctor may suggest trying one or more of these therapies as a first line of treatment. Behavior therapy may be the only treatment required. But these techniques can also be used before other types of treatment, such as medications or surgery, or in combination with them.

Fluid and diet management

How much fluid you drink and the types of food you eat may have an influence on your bladder habits. Too much fluid or too little fluid can trigger an overactive bladder, in which your bladder contracts and sends messages to your brain that it's full even when it's not. This can give you a strong urge to urinate or make you want to urinate more often, sometimes causing leakage as well. Occasionally, certain foods can irritate your bladder and increase frequency, urgency and leakage.

Too much fluid

It's true that drinking too much fluid can make you urinate more often. Particularly if you drink too much fluid at any one time, it can overwhelm your bladder and create a strong sense of urgency. If you exercise a lot or work outdoors on a regular basis, you may need to take in additional fluids. But rather than drink a large amount at once, try to spread your intake throughout the day.

If you get up several times a night to urinate, keep most of your fluid intake to the morning and afternoon and eliminate alcohol and caffeinated beverages and foods. In general, aim for about 8 cups of fluid a day. Remember that this can come from any beverage you drink, not just water, and also from foods such as soup. According to the Institute of Medicine's guideline for water intake, letting your thirst be your guide typically gives you an adequate amount of fluid, both from drinks and food. It's recommended that if you're experiencing incontinence, you try to drink between 6 and $7 1/2$ cups of fluid a day.

Too little fluid

Surprisingly, drinking too little fluid also can cause problems. Too little fluid may cause your urine to become overly concentrated with your body's waste products. Highly concentrated urine is dark yellow and has a strong smell. It can irritate your bladder, increasing the urge and frequency with which you need to go. Concentrated urine can also lead to a urinary tract infection, which can in itself lead to symptoms of urge incontinence.

Bladder irritants

Certain foods and beverages can irritate your bladder as well. Caffeine and alcohol both act as diuretics, which means that they increase urine production. This can lead to increased frequency and urgency of urination.

Consuming too many acidic fruits and fruit juices (oranges, grapefruits, lemons, limes), spicy foods, tomato-based products, carbonated drinks, and foods that contain artificial sweeteners also may irritate your bladder, although why these foods sometimes cause irritation isn't exactly understood.

If caffeine or alcohol or one of these other foods is a regular part of your diet, you might try eliminating it for about a week to see if your symptoms improve. Cut out only one food or beverage at a time so that you can tell which one is causing the problem. You might not even have to eliminate your favorite foods entirely. Simply cutting down on the amount you consume may help. See the Appendix on page 188 for a list of dietary bladder irritants.

Bladder training

When you have an overactive bladder, you can become accustomed to urinating frequently or at the slightest urge. Sometimes, you may go to the bathroom even if you don't have the urge but you want to avoid a possible accident. After a while, your bladder begins sending "full" messages to your brain even when it's not full, and you feel compelled to go. Normally, you'd urinate six or seven times a day, with your bladder holding 6 to 12 ounces at a time. With overactive bladder, you may urinate 13 or more times a day and more than twice a night, all in small amounts.

Bladder training, or retraining, involves teaching your bladder new habits by urinating on a set schedule. This allows you to gain control over urges and your bladder to fill up properly. Such training can be helpful for men and women who have urge and other types of incontinence. A bladder-training program can be used alone or in combination with other therapies. It usually follows these basic steps:

Find out your pattern. For a few days, record in a bladder diary every time you urinate. For example, you may find that you tend to urinate every hour on the hour. Your doctor can then use this diary to help you establish a schedule for your bladder training.

Set your bathroom intervals. After you've discovered how much time typically passes between bathroom breaks, your doctor will likely suggest you extend that interval by 15 minutes. So, if you determine that your usual interval is one hour, you work to extend that interval to an hour and 15 minutes.

Stick to your schedule. Once you've established a daytime schedule (you probably won't need to follow a schedule at night), do your best to stick to it. This is where your active participation comes in. Start out your schedule by urinating immediately after you wake up in the morning. Thereafter, if an urge arises but it's not time for you to go, try as hard as you can to wait it out. If you feel that you're going to have an accident, go to the bathroom but then return to your preset schedule.

Urges typically build to a peak and then gradually go away. Responding immediately to an urge by rushing to the bathroom only serves to increase your sense of urgency and may even invite an accident. Instead, stop and take a deep breath. Relax and try to think of something other than going to the bathroom. Play a mind game such as recalling the last three books you've read or the movies you've been meaning to watch. It may help to do a few quick pelvic floor muscle contractions (described below) to maintain control. Even if you feel an urge to go at your scheduled time, stop and wait until the urge recedes, then proceed slowly to the bathroom.

Increase your intervals. The goal is to gradually lengthen the time between trips to the bathroom until you reach intervals of two to four hours. You might do this by extending your intervals an additional 15 minutes each week until you reach the desired goal.

Don't be discouraged if you don't succeed the first few times. Keep practicing, and your ability to maintain control is very likely to increase. See the Appendix on page 198 for instructions on performing timed voiding drills.

Pelvic floor muscle training

Pelvic floor muscle training involves doing exercises, commonly referred to as Kegels, to strengthen weak urinary sphincter and pelvic floor muscles — the muscles that help control urination and defecation. The pelvic floor muscles serve dual roles. One is to open and close the urethra and anus. The other is to support the bladder and rectum — like a muscular sling — as you exert yourself doing everyday activities such as walking, standing, lifting and sneezing. The pelvic floor muscles stretch between your legs and attach to the front, back and sides of your pelvic bone. Your doctor may recommend that you exercise these muscles three or four times a day to treat your incontinence. These exercises are especially effective for women with stress incontinence, but can also help reduce or eliminate urge incontinence. See the Appendix on page 191 for information about how to perform pelvic floor exercises.

Biofeedback

A technique called biofeedback can help you with your pelvic floor muscle exercises, particularly if you're having trouble feeling or sensing these muscles. Biofeedback is a system that uses a variety of monitoring procedures and equipment to provide you with feedback on bodily responses such as muscle activity, heart rate, skin temperature and brain electrical activity. Using this information, you can learn to control some of these bodily responses to improve your health.

In the case of urinary incontinence, biofeedback can be used to monitor the electrical activity of your pelvic floor muscles and make sure you're using the right muscles when you do pelvic floor exercises. Many trained specialists conduct biofeedback sessions. They include nurses, occupational therapists, physical therapists and psychologists. In addition, there are biofeedback devices you can use at home.

During a biofeedback session, you or your therapist inserts a small sensor in your vagina or rectum. Sometimes, sensors are placed in both areas. In some cases, sensors can't be placed internally and instead small electrodes are placed on the skin adjacent to the pelvic floor muscles. Electrodes may also be placed on your abdomen, thighs or buttocks to see if you're unintentionally using these muscles during a pelvic floor muscle contraction. Then you're asked to contract your pelvic floor muscles several times as the sensors register the strength and control of your contractions. By watching the readout and comparing your response with the ideal response, you can modify your contractions so that you're doing the exercises properly.

Hand-held electronic devices that you use at home to measure the strength of your pelvic floor muscle contractions (Liberty, Myself, Peritron, PFX) can be purchased at drugstores and medical supply stores. Not all of them require a prescription. If you're interested in using biofeedback at home, ask your doctor or therapist if one of these devices might be appropriate for you.

Electrical stimulation

Weak electrical current is sometimes used to treat the muscles and nerves that play a role in urinary incontinence. The current is applied through electrodes that are placed either near the muscles or directly into the nerves they're designed to treat.

Pelvic floor muscle stimulation. If your pelvic floor muscles are very weak or if you need help with your pelvic floor exercises, your doctor or therapist may suggest electrical pelvic stimulation. With electrical stimulation, electrodes are temporarily inserted into your rectum or vagina to gently stimulate and strengthen your pelvic floor muscles. The electrical stimulation causes your pelvic floor muscles to contract without effort on your part (passive contractions). Electrical stimulation can also be used with strengthening exercises for very weak muscles. This technique can be effective for stress and urge incontinence in both men and women, but it often takes several months and multiple treatments to work. The procedure may be done in your doctor's or therapist's office, or you can do it at home with a portable battery-operated device.

Tibial nerve stimulation. Inspired by acupuncture, this method of electrical stimulation is used specifically to treat urge incontinence. Rather than stimulating the pelvic muscles, it stimulates the tibial nerve located in your lower leg. The tibial nerve is connected to the sacral nerve group, which plays a direct role in regulating bladder contractions. Stimulation of the tibial nerve can help to moderate the imbalanced nerve messages an overactive bladder sends to the brain, reducing the number of bladder contractions and the symptoms of urgency and frequency.

Tibial nerve stimulation may be done in your doctor's office. During the procedure, a thin needle is inserted just above your anklebone. Low-frequency electrical stimulation is passed through the needle to your tibial nerve for approximately 30 minutes. The procedure is painless, but you might notice your toes spread out or your big toe curl. You may also feel a sensation spread through the sole of your foot. The stimulation is applied once a week for about three months and then as needed thereafter, depending on your response to the therapy.

Preliminary clinical trials have shown the therapy to substantially improve signs and symptoms of incontinence, particularly frequency and urgency. More studies are needed to examine the therapy's long-term effects. Tibial nerve stimulation may provide an attractive alternative for people who have exhausted other conservative methods and would rather not have surgery.

Sacral nerve stimulation. Direct stimulation of the sacral nerve, which branches off your lower spinal cord, is another option for treating overactive bladder. This therapy requires a surgical procedure and is discussed in Chapter 6.

Other lifestyle changes

You can make other changes in your daily habits, such as managing the medications you take, managing your weight, stopping smoking and treating constipation, that may improve your incontinence symptoms.

Managing your medications
Medications that you're taking for another medical condition may cause or contribute to incontinence. If you have problems with incontinence or difficulty urinating, talk to your doctor about the

medications you're taking. Your doctor may be able to suggest an alternative dosage or another medicine that may not cause these kinds of side effects.

Examples of drugs that may contribute to incontinence include high blood pressure drugs, heart medications, diuretics, muscle relaxants, sedatives and antidepressants. Common effects of these medications include:

- Relaxation of the urethral muscle, which can lead to leakage
- Relaxation of the bladder muscle, which can lead to urinary retention and overflow incontinence
- Diminishing your awareness of the need to urinate
- Overproduction of urine, which can overwhelm an already stressed bladder
- Constipation, which can obstruct urine flow and aggravate an overactive bladder
- Chronic coughing, which can worsen stress incontinence

See the Appendix on page 192 for a list of types of medications that may contribute to urinary incontinence.

Managing your weight

Being overweight also may contribute to urinary incontinence, particularly stress and mixed incontinence. This may be because excessive body weight increases pressure on your abdomen during

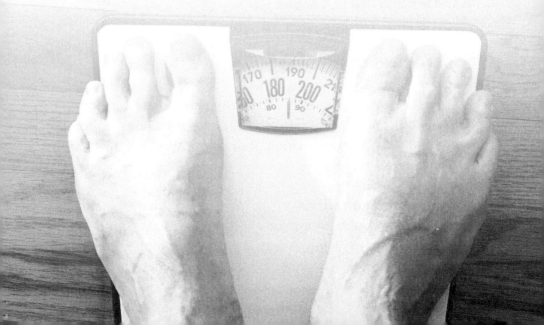

physical activity, which in turn may increase pressure on your bladder and the ability of your urethra to shift position, resulting in leakage. One study found that the risk of severe incontinence was three times as high for obese women as for normal-weight women. On the other hand, another study found that moderately obese women who lost as little as 5 percent of their body weight experienced an improvement in their symptoms. If you're overweight and are experiencing urinary incontinence, entering a weight-loss program may be one way to help treat your incontinence.

Stopping smoking

Smoking tobacco products is another lifestyle factor that may have an impact on urinary incontinence. Heavy smokers in particular tend to develop a severe chronic cough, which can place added pressure on the bladder and aggravate urinary incontinence. Stopping smoking allows your lungs to regain at least some normalcy, thus reducing or even eliminating your coughing and its effects on your bladder. Improving urinary incontinence may be one of many benefits of stopping smoking.

Your role in treatment

Behavior therapies can be very effective in the treatment of urinary incontinence and can provide substantial benefits with a minimum of side effects. Your doctor can help you in many ways — by teaching you how to implement different therapies, providing you with feedback and helping you manage your medications — but you also play a vital role in your treatment.

Once you learn how to do pelvic floor muscle exercises, for example, or begin a bladder-training program, your job is to actively carry out your prescribed treatment. Many behavior therapies take some time and practice before you begin seeing results. But persistence pays off. If you stick with the program, you'll more than likely see an improvement in your symptoms. And if one type of therapy doesn't work, talk with your doctor about exploring other options that may serve you better.

Finally, try to surround yourself with a positive network of family and friends. Although incontinence may be an embarrassing topic to discuss at first, you might be surprised at how common it really is. You may also discover how understanding others can be once they learn the implications of the condition and the benefits of its treatment, both for you and for them.

Chapter 5

Medications and devices for treating urinary incontinence

In some cases, your doctor may recommend one or more medications to treat your incontinence. Often, medications are taken in conjunction with behavior therapy.

In addition to medications, medical devices are available to help treat urinary incontinence, particularly in women. These devices may be worn to stop leakage or to hold up a weak bladder. Manual drainage procedures such as self-catheterization are another alternative for both men and women. These devices and procedures are discussed at the end of this chapter.

Medications

A number of drugs are used to treat all types of incontinence. Medications have been most helpful for people with overactive bladder. Stress incontinence is more often treated with behavior therapy such as pelvic floor muscle training, partly because behavior therapy produces satisfactory results in many people and partly because until now no specific medication existed for stress incontinence.

But new medications, both for stress incontinence and overactive bladder, are becoming available. These new medications are easier to take and have fewer side effects than the older ones. As a result, medications are becoming a more effective part of incontinence treatment than in the past.

When talking to your doctor, carefully review all of the medications you're taking for any other condition, including any over-the-counter drugs or herbal remedies. Some medications can worsen your incontinence, depending on what type you have. Others may interact with your incontinence medication in a way that increases your symptoms. Your doctor can help you decide what's best for you.

The major types of medications used to manage urinary incontinence include:

- Anticholinergics
- Estrogen
- Alpha-adrenergic blockers
- Alpha-adrenergic agonists

Other drugs also are used, including imipramine, an antidepressant, and desmopressin, a medication often used for bed-wetting in children.

Anticholinergics

If you could take a close look at the cells in your body, you would see tiny receptors on the outside surface of each cell. These receptors act as gateways for various chemical messengers (neurotransmitters) from the brain that tell your cells how to act. Each neurotransmitter fits a matching receptor, like a key in a lock.

Acetylcholine is a neurotransmitter that acts on bladder muscle cells to cause contractions of your bladder. Because overactive bladder is characterized by abnormal contractions, which make you want to urinate even when your bladder isn't full, anticholinergic drugs work by blocking the receptors to which acetylcholine normally binds (muscarinic receptors). This action has three results. It:

- Decreases involuntary bladder muscle contractions
- Reduces the strength of involuntary contractions
- Increases the storage capacity of your bladder

As a result, your bladder receives fewer unwanted messages to contract, and your urgency, frequency and incontinence episodes are diminished.

The two most commonly prescribed anticholinergics are oxybutynin (Ditropan) and tolterodine (Detrol). Both are available in an extended-release form, which has two advantages over the immediate-release forms. You only need to take them once a day instead of several times a day, and they have fewer side effects. Still, the immediate-release form may be helpful if you experience incontinence only at certain times, such as at night.

A study comparing the extended-release forms of oxybutynin and tolterodine found them to be similarly effective, although oxybutynin appeared to be slightly better at providing overall symptom relief. Side effects were generally mild.

Oxybutynin is also available as a skin patch that delivers a continuous amount of medication to your body for three and a half days. Initial studies have shown the skin patch to be as effective as the oral immediate-release form of oxybutynin, but with fewer side effects.

Propantheline (Pro-Banthine) and hyoscyamine (Levsin) have also been used to treat overactive bladder, but because of their pronounced side effects are no longer used as much.

Anticholinergics are the drugs of choice for women with overactive bladder. Research on anticholinergics for men has been limited by the fact that symptoms of overactive bladder often coincide or overlap with symptoms of an enlarged prostate (benign prostatic hyperplasia, or BPH). In this case the goal is to treat the enlarged prostate, which will then usually relieve your incontinence. If BPH or an obstruction such as a tumor isn't the cause of your bladder symptoms, your doctor may recommend treatment with an alpha-adrenergic blocker. If this doesn't work and surgery isn't an option for you, then you and your doctor may decide to try an anticholinergic, even though more research is needed to determine its effectiveness in men.

Side effects and cautions. The most common side effect of anticholinergics is dry mouth. To counteract this effect, you might suck on a piece of candy or chew gum to produce more saliva. Other less common side effects include constipation, heartburn, blurry vision, urinary retention and cognitive side effects such as dizziness and confusion.

The most common side effect of the oxybutynin skin patch is skin irritation. Your doctor may recommend that you rotate the location of your patch so that you use the same site only every other week.

Do not take an anticholinergic if you have problems with urinary retention, gastrointestinal obstruction or uncontrolled narrow-angle glaucoma. Use anticholinergics with caution if you have liver or kidney problems.

Estrogen

A woman's bladder and urethra also contain receptors for the hormone estrogen. Estrogen helps maintain the strength and flexibility of tissues in this area. After menopause, a woman's body produces less estrogen. The theory is that this drop in estrogen contributes to the deterioration of the supportive tissues around the bladder and urethra, which makes these tissues weak and eventually leads to stress incontinence.

Estrogen is known to improve blood flow, enhance nerve function and correct tissue deterioration in the bladder and vaginal areas. Applying estrogen in the form of a vaginal cream, ring or patch may help tone and rejuvenate these areas and relieve some of the symptoms of stress incontinence. Oral estrogen may not have the same benefits as topical creams and ointments.

In general, there's not a lot of scientific evidence to support the use of estrogen for treating urinary incontinence. A number of studies have found estrogen to be not much better than a placebo, although it may have a role when used in combination with other therapies, such as pelvic floor muscle training.

Side effects and cautions. The Women's Health Initiative — a large study sponsored by the National Institutes of Health — found that taking combination hormone replacement therapy (estrogen plus progestin) can rarely increase serious health risks, such as for heart disease, stroke, breast cancer and dementia. In addition, a large study of hormone replacement therapy and cardiovascular health found that taking combination hormone replacement therapy may actually worsen urinary incontinence.

In light of this evidence, combination hormone replacement therapy generally isn't prescribed for urinary incontinence and is only advised when its benefits outweigh its risks. On the other hand, estrogen in the form of a vaginal cream or ring has a much more localized effect than does the oral form and not as much of it enters your bloodstream. As a result it's not likely to produce the overall risks associated with oral hormone therapy.

Alpha-adrenergic blockers

These drugs were originally developed to treat high blood pressure, but they're also used to treat prostate enlargement in men and have been found to improve symptoms of overactive bladder and overflow incontinence. Alpha-adrenergic blockers, also known as alpha blockers, promote the relaxation of smooth muscle in your bladder neck and urethra by blocking the neurotransmitter norepinephrine from binding with alpha-adrenergic receptors in these areas. This tends to increase flow — the amount of urine you pass each time you urinate — and to decrease frequency — the number of times you need to urinate.

Your doctor may recommend one of these drugs if you're having symptoms of overactive bladder, even if you don't have an obstruction of the bladder, such as an enlarged prostate in men. The true effect of these drugs for overactive bladder is difficult to ascertain because most clinical trials have studied symptoms of overactive bladder and obstruction together, making it hard to distinguish the effect of each drug's separate and specific effect on overactive bladder.

Examples of alpha-adrenergic blockers include:
- Tamsulosin (Flomax)
- Alfuzosin (Uroxatral, Xatral)
- Doxazosin (Cardura)
- Terazosin (Hytrin)
- Prazosin (Minipress)

Side effects and cautions. Alpha-adrenergic blockers can cause a sudden drop in blood pressure when you change from one position to another, such as getting up from bed or standing up from a chair (postural hypotension). This may be particularly true when they're taken with drugs for impotence, such as sildenafil (Viagra), vardenafil (Levitra) or tadalafil (Cialis).

To reduce your risk of side effects, your doctor may start out with a low dose of the alpha blocker and gradually increase the dosage to an optimum point for you. If you're already taking a blood pressure medication (antihypertensive), your doctor may wish to monitor you for side effects.

Alpha-adrenergic agonists

Alpha-adrenergic agonists do the opposite of alpha-adrenergic blockers. Instead of blocking the alpha-adrenergic receptors in the bladder neck and urethra, these drugs stimulate the receptors by mimicking the action of norepinephrine. This has the effect of contracting the urethral smooth muscle, thus tightening the urinary sphincter and preventing urine from leaking out.

Examples of alpha-adrenergic agonists include ephedrine, pseudoephedrine and the now-discontinued phenylpropanolamine (PPA). These drugs aren't designed specifically for incontinence, but ephedrine and pseudoephedrine are commonly found in over-the-counter cough medicines, antihistamines and appetite suppressants. Although these drugs may be helpful for mild cases of stress incontinence, their use in such cases has decreased because of potentially dangerous side effects.

Side effects and cautions. The Food and Drug Administration (FDA) requested in 2000 that drug companies discontinue marketing products containing PPA after a study found that it increased the risk of stroke, particularly in women. It's possible that ephedrine and pseudoephedrine may have similar effects, so these drugs should be used with caution.

Side effects include agitation, insomnia, anxiety, dry mouth and headache. Avoid the use of alpha-adrenergic agonists if you have glaucoma, diabetes, hyperthyroidism, heart disease or high blood pressure.

Other drugs

Some drugs don't fall into any of the above categories but are still used as part of the arsenal of medications for urinary incontinence.

Imipramine. Imipramine (Tofranil) is a tricyclic antidepressant that has both anticholinergic and alpha-adrenergic effects. It causes the bladder muscle to relax, while causing the smooth muscles at the bladder neck to contract. As such, it may be used to treat mixed — urge and stress — incontinence. Because it causes drowsiness, it may improve nighttime incontinence, as well. It may also be helpful for children who bed-wet at night (nocturnal enuresis).

Imipramine can cause serious side effects involving the cardiovascular system, such as postural hypotension and irregular heartbeat. Children may be especially susceptible to these side effects. Other side effects, including dry mouth, blurry vision and constipation, are similar to those of anticholinergics. Tricyclic antidepressants interact with many different medications, so make sure your doctor knows which medications you're taking before you begin taking imipramine.

Desmopressin. Desmopressin is a synthetic version of a natural body hormone called anti-diuretic hormone (ADH). This hormone slows the production of urine. Your body normally produces more ADH at night, so the need to urinate is lower then.

In children, nocturnal enuresis may be caused by a shortage of nighttime production of ADH. Desmopressin is commonly used to treat nocturnal enuresis in children and is available as a nasal spray or pill for use before bedtime.

Two studies have suggested that desmopressin may also reduce nighttime incontinence in adult men and women. Side effects are uncommon, but there is a risk of water retention and sodium deficiency in the blood (hyponatremia), particularly in older adults.

Drugs under development

The old view of incontinence as an inevitable part of aging is changing. Pads and absorbent products are no longer seen as the mainstay of treatment. Instead, physicians and patients are pursuing better ways of treating urinary incontinence so that it doesn't inhibit quality of life. One result of this approach is the research and development of new drugs that may have longer lasting benefits and fewer side effects. Here are some examples:

Duloxetine. Duloxetine is a new drug with conditional approval for treating depression but which is also being evaluated specifically for treating stress incontinence.

Duloxetine is in a class of drugs called selective serotonin and norepinephrine reuptake inhibitors (SNRIs). These drugs interact with the neurotransmitters serotonin and norepinephrine. They are selective because they work almost exclusively on serotonin and norepinephrine and have little effect on other neurotransmitters.

When a nerve cell sends a message to another nerve cell via neurotransmitters, it releases the neurotransmitters into a gap (synapse) between the sending cell and the receiving cell. After the neurotransmitters have connected to their appropriate receptors on the receiving cell, they return to the sending cell. This process is called reuptake.

Duloxetine works by inhibiting the reuptake of serotonin and norepinephrine. This keeps the neurotransmitters in the synapse for a longer time, where they remain active and continue triggering messages. One of the effects of this action is to promote relaxation of the bladder muscle and increase the strength of the bladder outlet (urethral sphincter), thus increasing bladder storage capacity while reducing or preventing leakage.

During several controlled, randomized trials, duloxetine significantly improved incontinence in women, as opposed to a placebo. In most of the studies, quality of life also improved. The most common side effect of the drug is nausea, but it's usually mild and goes away in a few weeks.

Although duloxetine is being developed primarily to treat stress incontinence, it may also be helpful for mixed incontinence. While available abroad, the drug has yet to be approved for treating incontinence in the United States.

Selective anticholinergics. One of the limitations of current anticholinergic drugs is that they interact with a number of receptors throughout the body, such as the salivary glands and central nervous systems, in addition to those in the bladder. This produces a greater range of side effects, such as dry mouth and dizziness.

Darifenacin (Enablex), solifenacin (Vesicare) and trospium (Sanctura) are three recently approved anticholinergics that target specific receptors in the bladder muscle in order to treat overactive bladder. By being selective in the receptors with which they interact, these drugs may produce fewer side effects than do drugs like oxybutynin (Ditropan) and tolterodine (Detrol) while providing the same benefits.

Capsaicin and resiniferatoxin. Some studies have shown that capsaicin, the spicy component of hot chili peppers, has an anesthetizing effect on hypersensitive bladders. After the bladder is filled (instilled) with the capsaicin extract by means of a catheter, the extract at first stimulates the sensory nerves of the bladder and then produces a long-term resistance to sensory activation, which may last for two to seven months. Capsaicin has been used successfully as a treatment for overactive bladder associated with nerve disorders (neurogenic disorders) such as multiple sclerosis or traumatic spinal injuries.

Temporary side effects include discomfort and a burning sensation in the pubic area when the capsaicin is instilled. Instilling lidocaine before the capsaicin can help alleviate this problem.

Resiniferatoxin is an extract from a cactus-like plant and has effects similar to capsaicin. It is a thousand times as potent as capsaicin but doesn't produce any burning sensations in the pubic area when instilled into the bladder. In addition, studies of resiniferatoxin have found that it doesn't produce the temporary worsening of bladder symptoms that's seen with capsaicin, and its beneficial effects may last up to three months.

In clinical trials, resiniferatoxin has been successful in treating overactive bladder associated with neurogenic disorders, but the same benefits for non-neurogenic overactive bladder have yet to be seen.

Botulinum toxin type A. Injections of botulinum toxin type A (Botox) into the bladder muscle have benefited people who have an overactive bladder associated with nerve damage (neuropathic bladder overactivity), such as people with a spinal cord injury or children born with spina bifida.

Botox has the effect of blocking the actions of acetylcholine and paralyzing the bladder muscle. The injection is done through a long, slender instrument that carries a small camera at its tip by which your doctor can view the inside of your bladder (cystoscope).

Preliminary studies have found that Botox significantly improves symptoms of incontinence and causes very few side

Medications used to treat urinary incontinence

Medication	Type of incontinence	People who are likely to benefit
Anticholinergics • Darifenacin (Enablex) • Hyoscyamine (Cystospaz, Levsin) • Oxybutynin (Ditropan) • Propantheline (Pro-Banthine) • Propiverine* • Solifenacin (Vesicare) • Tolterodine (Detrol) • Trospium (Sanctura)	Overactive bladder	Mostly women
Estrogen • Vaginal cream (Estrace, Premarin) • Vaginal ring (Estring)	Overactive bladder	Women
Alpha-adrenergic blockers • Alfuzosin (Uroxatral, Xatral) • Doxazosin (Cardura) • Prazosin (Minipress) • Tamsulosin (Flomax) • Terazosin (Hytrin)	Overactive bladder Overflow incontinence	Men
Alpha-adrenergic agonists • Pseudoephedrine (Claritin-D, Chlor-Trimeton, Sudafed, others)	Stress incontinence	Men and women
Imipramine (Tofranil)	Overactive bladder Stress incontinence Mixed incontinence Nighttime incontinence	Men and women
Desmopressin (DDAVP)	Bed-wetting Nighttime incontinence	Mostly children but possibly also men and women

*Currently not available in the United States.

effects. Benefits last from six to nine months. In a study of 15 children with overactive bladder caused by spina bifida, 13 became completely dry after being treated with Botox. Other studies have found that Botox significantly reduced the need for medications and catheterization in people with neuropathic overactive bladder. When compared with resiniferatoxin, Botox appeared to provide superior benefits.

Scientists speculate that Botox may also be helpful for people with severe overactive bladder symptoms unrelated to a neurological condition, who haven't responded to other medications.

Medical devices

A number of medical devices are available that can help keep you dry or at least reduce leakage. Some of these devices can be put in and taken out at your discretion. Others can be worn all the time. Most devices are designed for women, but a few external devices are also available for men.

The benefit of these devices is that you control their use. Although they don't cure incontinence, they can help you manage it. The downside is that, for some people, some of these devices can be uncomfortable and even painful. If you have questions, ask your doctor. He or she can help you decide if one of these medical devices would be helpful for you.

Urethral inserts

Urethral inserts are small, tampon-like disposable devices or plugs that a woman inserts into her urethra to prevent urine from leaking out. Urethral inserts aren't for everyday use. They work best for women who have predictable incontinence during certain activities, such as while playing tennis. The device is inserted before the activity. Whenever the woman needs to urinate, she simply removes the device. Urethral inserts are available by prescription.

One example of a urethral insert is the FemSoft Insert. The single-use, disposable device — made of soft silicone — is shaped like a tube with a balloon-like tip at one end and a flange at the other.

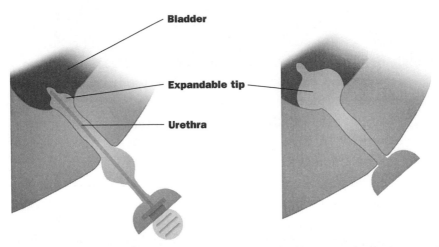

Bladder

Expandable tip

Urethra

The FemSoft Insert is placed in a woman's urethra where it forms a barrier between the bladder and the outside, thus preventing the leakage of urine during activities that might otherwise cause incontinence.

Encasing the tube is a sheath filled with mineral oil. After the device is inserted into the bladder with an applicator, most of the fluid blows into the balloon tip. Because the balloon tip is soft and fluid-filled, it conforms to the shape of your bladder and creates a seal around your bladder neck, preventing urine from leaking out. To remove the insert, you grasp the flange, which remains on the outside of your urethra, and pull the device out.

Pessary

Your doctor may prescribe a pessary (PES-uh-re) — a silicone or latex device, usually shaped like a ring or a dish, that's inserted into your vagina and that you can wear all day. The device helps hold up your bladder, which lies near the vagina, to prevent urine leakage. You may benefit from a pessary if you have incontinence due to a dropped (prolapsed) bladder or uterus.

A pessary is usually fitted and put in place by your doctor. If you have an infection in your pelvic area, it must be treated before you are fitted with the device, to avoid complications. You don't always need to remove it to urinate, but you do need to regularly remove it to clean it. Some of the side effects that can occur include an allergic reaction to the latex or silicone, infection and pressure sores. Pressure sores are more common if you're postmenopausal, most likely because vaginal tissue is typically more sensitive and less elastic after menopause. Vaginal estrogen cream may help in this case.

External barriers

Devices that are worn externally are available for women and men. These devices come in a variety of shapes and are designed to stop the flow of urine.

For women. Disposable, self-adhesive foam pads (Miniguard, UroMed, Impress Softpatch) are available that adhere to your urethral opening and stop urine from leaking. The pads are about the size of a postage stamp and fit in between your labia. You remove the pad to urinate and then insert a new one.

Another type of external barrier is a silicone cap (Bard CapSure, FemAssist) that fits over your urethral opening and uses suction to stay in place. It can be washed with soap and water and reused for up to one week.

For men. Penile clamps and compression rings are two devices available for men. The penile clamp fits over your penis. Its tightness can be adjusted to stop the flow of urine. The Cunningham clamp, which is used most often, has a foam cushion on the inside and a metal casing on the outside. The compression ring is inflated around the penis and also works by pinching off the flow of urine.

These devices should not be worn for more than two to three hours at a time. If left on for too long, they can cause tissue damage, swelling and pain.

Catheters

If other treatments fail or are unacceptable, or if you need help while waiting for a treatment such as surgery, your doctor may recommend that you use a catheter. A catheter is a thin tube that's placed in your urethra to allow you to drain your bladder manually. This may be done for you or you can learn to do it yourself. In some cases, the catheter may be left in. The catheter is connected to an external bag to hold urine. The bag is emptied as needed.

If you have nerve damage or you're a man with bladder problems resulting from an enlarged prostate, using a catheter at regular intervals can help empty your bladder completely and prevent overflow incontinence.

Common side effects of using a catheter include urinary tract infections and skin irritation. Careful use of sterile techniques while using the catheter can help you avoid these problems.

For men, there's also an external drainage system called a condom catheter, which fits over your penis like a condom and collects urine. The urine is then drained through a tube to a bag that's attached to your leg. Condom catheters come in disposable and reusable forms. An advantage of the condom catheter is that it doesn't require an internal catheter to be placed in your urethra. As a result, urinary tract infections are less common, although skin irritation may occur due to friction between the catheter and your penis.

Chapter 6

Surgical options for treating urinary incontinence

If behavior therapies and medications aren't working for you, your doctor may suggest one of a number of surgical options available to treat urinary incontinence. In general, surgery is reserved for when your symptoms haven't responded to other types of treatment and your incontinence is markedly disrupting your way of life.

Surgery is more invasive and has a higher risk of complications than other therapies, but it can also be effective in treating urinary incontinence and provide a long-term solution in severe cases. Most surgical options are used to treat stress incontinence, although surgical alternatives are now available for severe urge incontinence as well.

Things to know before surgery

Before you choose surgery to treat your incontinence, it's important to have an accurate diagnosis, because different types of surgery are used to treat different types of incontinence. Your doctor may refer you to an incontinence specialist, such as a urologist or urogynecologist, for further diagnostic testing. Tests may include cystourethroscopy, urinary tract imaging and urodynamic studies. (For more on these tests, see Chapter 3.)

If your incontinence is caused by a separate medical condition, treatment is aimed at correcting that condition, which may also resolve your incontinence. For example, if you're a man with overflow incontinence, surgery may be necessary to treat an enlarged prostate gland that's constricting the urethra. If you're a woman with incontinence caused by your bladder or uterus slipping out of position (pelvic organ prolapse), a surgeon may reposition the organ with one of a variety of techniques. Surgery might also be an option if you have incontinence caused by a tumor in the bladder or a uterine fibroid. In some cases, pregnancy or birthing injuries may need repair. Rarely, surgery to treat urinary incontinence may involve enlarging the bladder or correcting a birth defect.

As with any surgical procedure, surgery for urinary incontinence has the potential for complications such as bleeding, wound infection and organ injury, but these are uncommon. More frequently, urinary tract infection may occur after the operation, particularly if temporary catheterization is required. But this can be easily treated with antibiotics.

Although surgery almost always improves urinary incontinence, in some cases it may not completely cure your incontinence. In addition, surgery can only correct the problem it's designed to treat. If you have mixed incontinence, surgery for stress incontinence will not help urge incontinence, and you may need to take medications after surgery to address the urge incontinence. It's also possible that after surgery, urinary and genital problems may develop that previously didn't exist, including:

- Difficulty urinating and incomplete emptying of the bladder (urinary retention), although this is usually temporary
- Development of an overactive bladder, which could lead to urge incontinence
- Pelvic organ prolapse
- Difficult or painful intercourse

Talking with your surgeon before the operation can give you a good idea of the risks and benefits associated with the different types of surgery and help you decide which one may be best for your particular situation. For example, you may prefer a surgery with the lowest risk of complications or the shortest recovery time, or you may opt for one that gives you the greatest chance of a complete cure. In addition, your surgeon's experience is likely to play a role in the type of surgery you choose.

Surgery for urinary incontinence is rarely urgent. Furthermore, the success of treatment tends to decline with repeat surgeries. So, unless your doctor says otherwise, take your time learning about your options and reviewing them with your doctor or surgeon. This way, you'll be able to make the decision that's most likely to leave you satisfied with the results.

Surgery for stress incontinence

There are two types of stress incontinence. One is due to weakened pelvic floor muscle support of the bladder, bladder neck and urethra. Weakened support allows the bladder neck and urethra to temporarily shift position under physical pressure, such as when you cough or laugh, causing leakage of urine from the bladder. This condition is referred to as urethral hypermobility and is the most common cause of stress incontinence in women.

The second type of stress incontinence is caused by weakened or damaged urethral sphincter muscles that aren't able to properly seal off the urine in the bladder. This is termed intrinsic sphincteric deficiency (ISD).

These two conditions aren't related to each other, but you can have both at the same time. Procedures used when making your diagnosis should reveal whether your incontinence is caused primarily by urethral hypermobility or ISD. This knowledge is important in deciding which surgery to choose.

Several procedures have been developed to treat urethral hypermobility, all with the same goal — strengthening the urethra's support system. Most tend to fall into two main categories — bladder neck suspension procedures and sling procedures.

For ISD, the goal of treatment is to restore normal function of your urethral sphincter. Sling procedures are generally more effective than suspension procedures in treating ISD. Other treatments for ISD include artificial sphincters and injection with bulking agents.

Bladder neck suspension procedures

Bladder neck suspension procedures have traditionally been the surgery of choice in women with stress incontinence. These procedures are designed to support your bladder neck and urethra. The most common procedure performed is retropubic suspension. Needle suspension, also known as transvaginal suspension, has been an alternative in the past but is rarely used anymore.

Retropubic suspension. To do a retropubic suspension procedure, your surgeon makes a 3- to 5-inch incision in your lower abdomen. Through this incision, he or she places stitches (sutures) in the tissue near the bladder neck and secures the stitches to a liga-

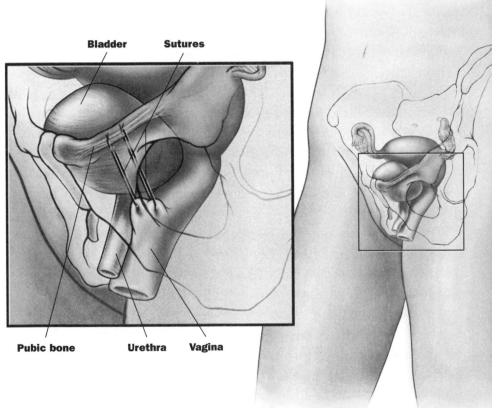

Bladder neck suspension surgery is aimed at adding support to the bladder neck and urethra, reducing the risk of stress incontinence. The procedure shown here is the Burch retropubic suspension. It involves placing sutures in vaginal tissue near the neck of the bladder (where the bladder and urethra meet) and attaching them to ligaments near the pubic bone.

ment near your pubic bone (Burch procedure) or in the cartilage of the pubic bone itself (Marshall-Marchetti-Krantz, or MMK, procedure). This has the effect of bolstering your urethra and bladder neck so that they don't sag.

Retropubic suspension is generally recommended as the procedure that produces the longest lasting chances of a cure for stress incontinence. Approximately 80 percent of women who undergo this procedure are cured for at least four years, and about 90 percent experience improvement.

The downside of this procedure is that it involves major abdominal surgery. It's done under general anesthesia and usually takes

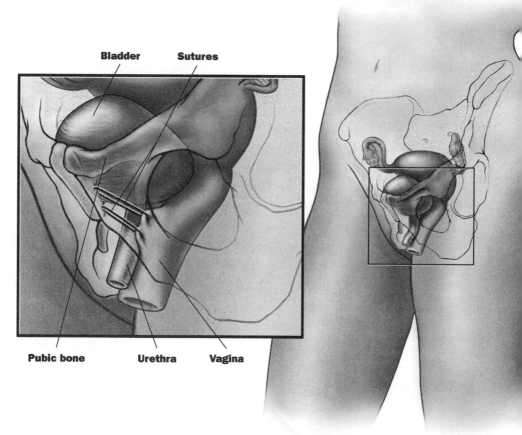

The Marshall-Marchetti-Krantz (MMK) retropubic bladder suspension procedure shown here is similar to the Burch procedure. In the MMK procedure, sutures are placed in vaginal tissue near the bladder neck and along the urethra and then secured to cartilage of the pubic bone.

about an hour. Recovery takes about six weeks, and you'll likely need to use a catheter until you can urinate normally.

The Burch procedure may also be done by inserting narrow, tube-like instruments through small incisions in the abdomen (laparoscopy). Long-term studies haven't confirmed the therapeutic benefits of this approach and, as a result, many surgeons have stopped using it.

Needle suspension. Needle (transvaginal) suspension has a higher risk of failure and a lower long-term cure rate — around 67 percent — than does retropubic suspension. Most urogynecologists and urologists don't recommend needle suspension procedures except in rare circumstances. To do this procedure, a surgeon uses incisions in the vagina to place supportive stitches around the bladder neck and urethra. After the stitches are placed through the vaginal incisions, they're passed through a tiny abdominal incision and attached to the abdominal wall or pelvic bone.

Sling procedures

Rather than using stitches to bolster the neck of the bladder, sling procedures use strips of tissue or synthetic tape that create a pelvic sling or hammock around your bladder neck and urethra. The sling provides the support necessary to keep the urethra closed even when you cough or sneeze.

The procedure is most often used in women to treat stress incontinence and appears to be just as effective as retropubic suspension, with a cure rate of around 80 percent and an improvement rate of about 90 percent. Recent information shows that the sling is ineffective for male stress incontinence.

In a conventional sling procedure, the surgeon inserts a sling through a vaginal incision and brings it around the bladder neck. The sling is most often made of a synthetic tape, though occasionally your own tissue or animal tissue may be used. The ends of the sling are brought through a small abdominal incision and adjusted to achieve the right amount of tension. The ends are then attached to pelvic tissue (fascia) or to the abdominal wall with stitches.

A more recent trend is to use tissue friction to hold a synthetic mesh tape in place. No stitches are used to attach the mesh sling.

Instead, tissue itself holds the sling in place and eventually scar tissue forms in and around the tape to keep it from moving.

Sling procedures are less invasive than retropubic bladder neck suspension procedures, they don't take as long, and they can be done under local anesthesia on an outpatient basis. The advantage of having local anesthesia is that the surgeon can adjust the tension of the sling while you're awake by asking you to cough. This minimizes the risk of overtightening the sling, which can lead to urinary retention and prolonged catheterization after the operation. In addition, because of the instrumentation used, the tension-free sling allows for less cutting at the neck of the bladder.

The two variations on the tension-free sling are the retropubic technique and the transobturator technique.

Retropubic technique. This procedure, also referred to as a tension-free vaginal sling procedure, uses three small incisions: a vaginal incision and two abdominal incisions just above the pubic bone. With the help of a special needle, your surgeon threads one end of the tape through the vaginal incision, behind the pubic bone (retropubic space) and up through one of the abdominal incisions. Then, using a second needle, the surgeon passes the other end of the tape in the same manner up to the second abdominal incision, so that the tape forms a mesh hammock under the urethra. This process typically takes less than 30 minutes.

Once the tape is in place, your surgeon will ask you to cough. Your bladder will have been filled with fluid during the surgery, so your surgeon can tell if coughing still makes it leak. After adjusting the tape to an optimum tension, where only a drop or two of fluid leaks out, the surgeon snips the ends of the tape just under the surface of your skin and closes the incisions.

The disadvantage of this procedure is that the needles are passed blindly through the retropubic space and may possibly damage blood vessels, nerves, the bladder or the intestines. To make sure that the bladder hasn't been perforated, periodic viewing of the bladder's interior is done through a cystoscope, a tube-like instrument with a tiny video camera at its tip, that's passed up through the urethra into the bladder.

Retropubic

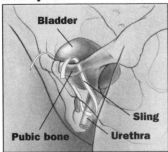

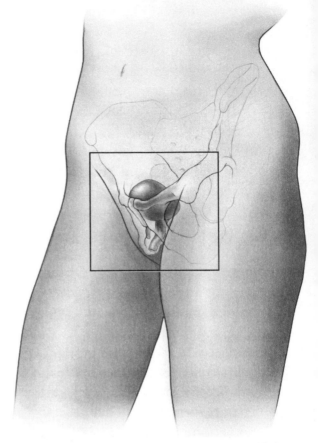

Transobturator

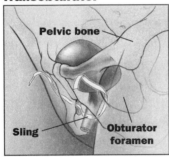

A sling is a piece of tissue or a synthetic tape that is surgically placed to support the bladder neck and urethra. Two sling techniques are shown — the retropubic and transobturator. Both are designed to reduce or eliminate stress incontinence in women.

Transobturator technique. The transobturator procedure theoretically carries a lower risk of injury than does the retropubic technique because the needles and tape are passed via the obturator foramen, a pair of openings on either side of the pelvic area, rather than behind the pubic bone (retropubic area). The obturator space is thought to be anatomically safer than the retropubic area because it doesn't contain any major blood vessels and exposure to the bladder and other organs is limited. In addition, cystoscopy isn't always necessary for this procedure.

To do the transobturator technique, your surgeon makes small incisions on either side of your groin and passes a curved needle through the obturator foramen to a vaginal incision where one end of the tape is fastened to the needle. Carrying the tape, the needle is pulled back through the obturator foramen and out through the groin incision. The same process is repeated on the other side. Once the tape is in place under the urethra, a cough test is performed to make sure the tape is properly positioned. The surgeon then snips the ends of the tape and closes the incisions. The tape is held in place by friction between it and the surrounding tissue.

Recovery time for tension-free slings is fairly short — it's usually only a week or two before you're able to return to your regular activities. Because of the simplicity of this procedure, it's becoming the procedure of choice for treating stress incontinence in women.

Bulking agents

Compared with other surgical options, the use of bulking agents is relatively noninvasive and may be an option if you would rather not risk the complications of major surgery. Treatment with a bulking agent involves the injection of a material that adds bulk to the tissue surrounding the urethra next to the urethral sphincter. This serves to tighten the seal of the sphincter and stop urine from leaking. Bulking agents may be particularly useful for women with intrinsic sphincteric deficiency (ISD), a condition in which the urethral sphincter muscles don't seal off urine in the bladder, or men who've had their prostate removed. More recent evidence suggests that bulking agents may also help alleviate stress incontinence due to urethral hypermobility, a condition in which the bladder neck and urethra temporarily shift under pressure.

The bulking agent procedure is done with minimal anesthesia and typically takes about five minutes. For most women, the procedure can be done in a doctor's office. For men, the procedure is more involved because of anatomy, and is more often done in a hospital setting. The downside of most available bulking agents is that they lose their effectiveness over time and repeat injections are usually needed every six to 18 months.

New and improved bulking agents are being created, as well as new ways to make the injection process easier and more efficient. The standard method of injecting a bulking agent is through a needle, which is inserted several times in different positions with the

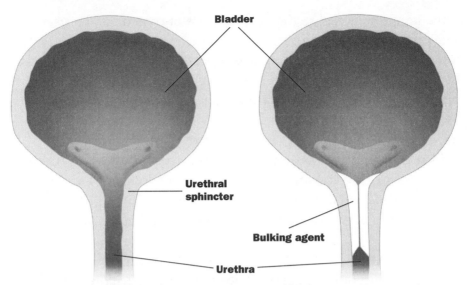

Bladder

Urethral
sphincter

Bulking agent

Urethra

Bulking agents are used to help tighten the area where urine flows from the bladder into the urethra. Bulking agents are injected into tissue next to the urethral sphincter to help prevent urine leakage.

assistance of a cystoscope, a slender, tube-like instrument that allows the surgeon to view the urethral area. This method requires great precision in order to place the needle in the correct spot and avoid injury to the urethral tissue. One of the newer methods not currently available in the United States uses predetermined needle positions to increase injection precision and eliminate the need for a cystoscope.

Following are some examples of bulking agents that are currently in use.

Collagen. Collagen (Contigen) is a natural fibrous protein found in connective tissue, bone and cartilage of humans and animals. Collagen obtained from cows is one of the most common bulking agents used. Collagen can produce an allergic reaction in some people. For this reason, your doctor is required to give you a skin test before performing the procedure to see if you have a reaction.

Short-term improvement rates after collagen injections range from around 60 percent to 85 percent. But over time the collagen tends to deteriorate within your body. After three years, the number of people whose symptoms remain improved decreases to 45 percent. Often, multiple repeat injections are required.

Carbon-coated zirconium beads. Carbon-coated zirconium beads (Durasphere) are among the synthetic bulking agents recently approved by the Food and Drug Administration (FDA). Durasphere has an advantage over some of the other synthetic agents in that its particles are big enough that they won't migrate. Durasphere is nonallergenic, which means it doesn't carry the risk of causing an adverse allergic reaction. A study comparing Durasphere and Contigen found them to be equally effective. Scientists hope that Durasphere will last much longer in the body than Contigen and require fewer repeat injections.

Ethylene vinyl alcohol copolymer. Ethylene vinyl copolymer (Tegress) was also recently approved by the FDA for use in treating stress incontinence. Tegress is injected in liquid form into the wall of the urethra near the bladder. Once in the body, Tegress absorbs water from surrounding tissues and solidifies into a spongy material. The spongy material adds bulk to the urethra, helping to prevent uncontrolled urination. The implant doesn't migrate, isn't absorbed by the body, and tissue grows into the material, helping to stabilize it. As with Contigen and Durasphere, Tegress is injected with cystoscopic guidance. About 75 percent of those who receive Tegress will require repeat injections.

Fat. Abdominal fat, withdrawn through liposuction, has also been used as a bulking agent. Its advantages are that it's readily available, and it's compatible with your body, so it isn't likely to cause an allergic reaction. However, a potential rare side effect is pulmonary embolism, in which a fat particle escapes and creates an obstruction in an artery in a lung. This condition can lead to severe respiratory problems and even death. When compared with collagen, fat appears to have a substantially lower cure rate. As a result, fat is rarely used as a bulking agent.

Note: The following bulking agents are not approved for use in the United States.

Dextranomer and hyaluronic acid copolymer (Zuidex, Deflux). Dextranomer and hyaluronic acid copolymer (Zuidex, Deflux), made in Sweden, has already been established as a treatment for vesicoureteral reflux (VUR), a condition in which urine in the bladder backs up into the ureters. (The ureters are a pair of ducts that carry urine from the kidney to the bladder.) Zuidex is now being evaluated in the United States as a treatment for stress incontinence. The advantages of Zuidex are that it doesn't migrate to other organs and it's nonallergenic. Growth of your own tissue into the material stabilizes it so that it doesn't deteriorate over time. A large, multicenter trial to study its effectiveness is under way.

Silicone. Silicone (Macroplastique) is a nonbiodegradable agent that consists of tiny rubber particles suspended in a type of gel. Some of these particles are so small that there's a possibility that they may migrate to other organs after injection. In addition, because silicone isn't biodegradable, there's a risk of granuloma formation. Granulomas are small masses or nodules of inflamed tissue that can migrate to other parts of the body. The success rate of silicone after 12 months has been reported to be about 50 percent to 60 percent. The manufacturers of Macroplastique have developed an injection procedure that doesn't require cystoscopic guidance.

Artificial sphincter

An artificial sphincter is a small device that's particularly helpful for men who have weakened urethral sphincters from treatment of prostate cancer or an enlarged prostate gland. It's rarely used for women with stress incontinence, unless they have severe incontinence due to ISD, and other treatments, including other types of surgery, haven't worked. In such cases, implantation of an artificial sphincter may be an option.

Surgery to place the device requires general or spinal anesthesia. The doughnut-shaped device is implanted around the neck of your bladder. Its fluid-filled ring keeps your urethral sphincter closed until you're ready to urinate. To urinate, you press a valve implanted under your skin that causes the ring to deflate and allows urine from your bladder to be released. Once your bladder is empty, the device reinflates over the next few minutes.

The pump isn't activated until sometime after the surgery so that the area has time to heal. For the first four to six weeks after surgery, you'll need to follow a few standard restrictions, such as no driving, no sexual activity, no strenuous activities and no sitting for long periods. In addition, you'll have some permanent restric-

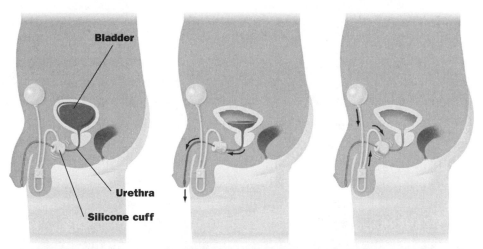

An artificial sphincter uses a small silicone cuff placed around the urethra to treat incontinence. When inflated, the cuff squeezes the urethra, preventing urine from leaking. To urinate, you deflate the cuff, allowing urine to pass.

tions, such as no riding bikes, motorcycles or other vehicles with a similar seat and no riding horses.

This surgery can cure or greatly improve incontinence in more than 70 percent to 80 percent of men with incontinence and in up to 90 percent of women. A potential disadvantage is that the device may malfunction, which means the surgery will need to be repeated.

Surgery for overactive bladder

Surgery for overactive bladder is generally considered a last resort. The majority of people with frequency and urgency problems and urge incontinence are treated with conservative therapies such as pelvic floor muscle training, bladder training, electrical stimulation and medications (see Chapters 4 and 5). But for men and women whose signs and symptoms are severe and who don't respond to these types of therapies, surgery may be an option.

Hydrodistention

Hydrodistention is sometimes used to treat overactive bladder. It's also a technique used to diagnose and temporarily treat inflammation of the bladder wall (interstitial cystitis). The effects of treating overactive bladder with hydrodistention are temporary and success rates vary widely.

Hydrodistention is performed by filling your bladder with fluid until it's stretched beyond its normal capacity, and allowing it to remain distended for several minutes. Stretching your bladder in this way can be painful, so the procedure is performed under general or local anesthesia, usually in a hospital. Most of the time, you're able to go home the same day.

Doctors aren't exactly sure how hydrodistention works, but the theory is that stretching the bladder wall serves to deaden overly sensitive nerve fibers, thus reducing the flow of sensory information between the bladder and the brain and decreasing the involuntary contractions characteristic of overactive bladder. People who've had it done report an improvement in their symptoms lasting around three months.

After the procedure, you may experience some pain in your pelvic area, especially when urinating the first few times. Your urine may contain some blood, but this is normal after the procedure. Discomfort may continue for a few weeks, but your doctor can prescribe pain relief medication to ease any pain or burning.

Potential complications of hydrodistention include bleeding, urinary retention and bladder perforation, although these are fairly uncommon. Another potential complication is interstitial fibrosis, which leads to stiffening of your bladder wall.

Sacral nerve stimulation

Your ability to urinate is governed by a complex set of voluntary and involuntary impulses between your brain and a nerve at the base of your spinal cord — the sacral nerve — that connects to your bladder. If this communication is disrupted or imbalanced, it can lead to an overactive bladder that sends too many impulses to your brain with the message that you need to urinate. This causes the strong urge characteristic of overactive bladder.

Sacral nerve stimulation seeks to inhibit these messages by continuously sending small, electrical impulses to the sacral nerve in your lower spine that controls urination. To do this, your surgeon places a thin wire with a small electrode tip near the sacral nerve.

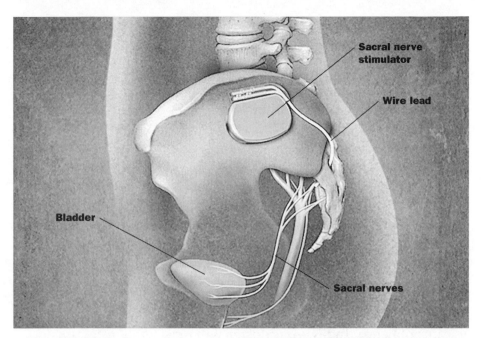

Sacral nerve stimulator

Wire lead

Bladder

Sacral nerves

The sacral nerve stimulator is an electronic device used to stimulate nerves that regulate bladder activity. The unit is placed beneath the skin of the buttocks, about where the back pocket is on a pair of pants. It's shown here out of place for a better view of the unit.

The wire is passed under your skin to a small, pacemaker-like device that's placed in a "pocket" of fat beneath the skin of your buttock just below the beltline. The device contains a special battery and electronics that control impulses to the sacral nerve.

Because the device doesn't work for everyone, your doctor can let you try it out first by wearing the device externally. If the stimulator substantially improves your symptoms, then you can have it implanted in your buttock. Surgery to implant the stimulator is done in an operating room under local anesthesia and usually involves recovery as an outpatient.

Once the stimulator is implanted, it runs for five to 10 years and can be replaced during an outpatient procedure. Your doctor can adjust the level of stimulation with a hand-held programmer.

The stimulation doesn't cause pain and may improve or cure 50 percent to 75 percent of people with difficult-to-treat urge incontinence or urinary retention leading to overflow incontinence. It's also an alternative to surgery to divert the urine or build a new bladder, which only helps 30 percent to 40 percent of the time.

Possible complications include infection. The device can be removed at any time.

If you're pregnant and wearing a stimulator, your doctor may advise you to turn it off as its effects on a fetus are unknown, although no problems have been reported. Because the stimulator is a metallic device, magnetic resonance imaging (MRI) isn't recommended because of the possibility of heating at the tip of the electrode, which can damage the nerve. There's also a 25 percent chance of ruining the battery.

Bladder augmentation

Bladder augmentation is an older procedure used to increase the size of your bladder. The operation is complex and involves major abdominal surgery. For a long time, it was the only procedure available for people with debilitating symptoms of frequency, urgency and incontinence. Today, your doctor will most likely recommend trying sacral nerve stimulation before bladder augmentation.

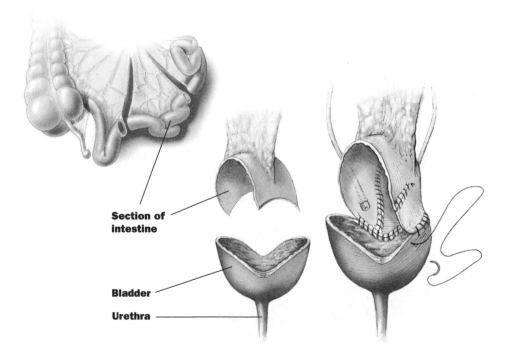

Section of intestine

Bladder

Urethra

Bladder augmentation takes tissue from the intestine or stomach and uses it to enlarge the size of the bladder, increasing its storage capacity.

To do bladder augmentation, your surgeon makes an incision in your abdomen and an opening at the top of your bladder. He or she then takes a strip of tissue, usually from your intestine or stomach, and attaches it onto the bladder opening. This added tissue patch increases the size of your bladder. The surgery is done under general anesthesia and may take several hours.

Recovery generally involves a stay at the hospital until you're able to start drinking and eating again. It usually takes a few weeks after you leave the hospital for you to return to your normal schedule. Many people, especially those with underlying nerve damage, require lifelong use of a catheter after the procedure.

Bladder augmentation doesn't always cure incontinence and can have complications such as infection and chronic diarrhea. Two rare but potentially serious complications are spontaneous perforation of the bladder and development of bladder cancer.

Urinary diversion

Under rare circumstances, such as when an overactive bladder is completely unresponsive to therapy or if all bladder function has been lost, urine may be stored and drained by means other than the bladder and urethra. This is called a urinary diversion.

Your surgeon creates a separate reservoir in your lower abdomen using a segment of your small intestine or colon. He or she then redirects your ureters to the reservoir so that the urine flows into it rather than your bladder. A small opening is made in your abdomen so that the urine can be drained into a bag or through a catheter.

Bladder denervation

A procedure called bladder denervation has also been done in which some or all of the nerves to the bladder are cut. This desensitizes the bladder in an effort to control pain and severe, chronic symptoms. When all of the nerves are cut, the bladder reflex is destroyed, and the urethral and anal sphincters cease to function, causing complete loss of bowel and urinary control. A few types of denervation procedures aim to spare some of the nerves in the bladder while helping to relieve pain. Denervation procedures rarely have helped people and are performed infrequently.

One step at a time

There are a wide variety of surgical procedures available for the treatment of urinary incontinence. They range from minimally invasive injection of bulking agents to major surgery. It's important to remember that if a particular treatment approach isn't working, there may be another solution to the problem. It's also important to keep in mind that finding an effective remedy may take time, with several steps along the way.

Chapter 7

Concerns specific to different groups

Although urinary incontinence can affect anyone — men and women, young and old — it's not the same for everyone. Men and women experience it differently, as do children and older adults. Basic anatomical and hormonal differences account for much of the difference between men and women. In women, urinary incontinence commonly results from weakened pelvic floor muscles, which may be caused by various life events and changes such as childbirth and menopause. In men weakened pelvic floor muscles usually aren't a problem, but problems associated with the prostate gland often contribute to urinary incontinence.

In children, the problem is frequently transient and gets better with time. In older adults, urinary incontinence may be associated with changes due to aging, the way in which the kidneys and bladder function, and various other risk factors, as well as diseases that become more common later in life, such as Parkinson's and Alzheimer's.

As a result, treatment may vary a little or a lot for different groups of people, depending on the nature of the underlying problem that's causing the incontinence. In this chapter we'll take a more detailed look at urinary incontinence from each of these perspectives and how management and treatment of incontinence may differ, depending on which group you fall into.

Women

Urinary incontinence is much more common in women than in men — in the under-65 age group, nearly seven times as many women as men experience it. Women may experience all types of urinary incontinence, but stress incontinence is most common.

Much of female urinary incontinence is due to wear and tear on a woman's reproductive system as a result of pregnancy, childbirth and hormonal changes associated with menopause. Physical changes resulting from these life events can lead to incontinence by weakening your pelvic floor muscles and the tissues supporting your urogenital area. Incontinence can also be associated with pelvic organ prolapse, a condition in which one of your pelvic organs, such as the bladder, slips through the vagina. Other less common causes of female incontinence include pelvic surgery and an abnormal connection between the vagina and the urethra (urethrovaginal urogenital fistula).

Pregnancy and childbirth

When you're pregnant, particularly during the last trimester, the increasing weight of your uterus places added pressure on the bladder and can result in stress incontinence. This type of incontinence is usually temporary and goes away after delivery.

In contrast, the stresses of labor and delivery can have a more lasting effect. Multiple births, prolonged difficult labors, forceps-assisted deliveries and perineal trauma such as tears or episiotomies can stretch the pelvic floor muscles and the ring of muscles that surround the urethra (urinary sphincter). Weakened pelvic floor muscles aren't always able to help keep the bladder neck closed tight, and this can lead to urine leakage when sudden increased pressure is placed on your bladder. The stress of childbearing can also damage nerves that lead to your bladder, and this can affect your bladder control. Incontinence may develop right after delivery or not until many years later.

In most women it generally takes about three months after delivery for pelvic floor muscles to regain their natural firmness and elasticity and for incontinence to improve. If you still experience leakage after six months, talk to your doctor about it so that you can be properly diagnosed and decide on a treatment plan. Without treatment, it may become a long-term problem. Treatment usually includes pelvic floor muscle training (Kegels) with or without biofeedback, and possibly electrical stimulation (see Chapter 4). Medications are also available to treat the problem (see Chapter 5). If your incontinence is severe, you and your doctor may consider surgical alternatives (see Chapter 6). If you're considering having more children, however, you may wish to postpone surgery until later, because gestation and delivery may cause recurrent incontinence following a successful operation.

You can take steps on your own to help prevent or improve incontinence associated with pregnancy and childbirth by doing Kegel exercises (see "Pelvic floor exercises" on page 191 to learn how these are done). Your pelvic floor muscles are just like other muscles in your body and can be toned and firmed with exercise. Doing Kegels regularly throughout your pregnancy and after delivery can strengthen your pelvic floor muscles and improve their effectiveness in keeping your bladder neck closed.

Pelvic organ prolapse

A condition called pelvic organ prolapse may be associated with stress incontinence and overactive bladder. Pelvic organ prolapse occurs when organs located in your pelvic area — your bladder, uterus, small intestine or rectum — fall or slip out of place (prolapse) and descend into the vagina. Often, pelvic organ prolapse produces no symptoms (that is, it's asymptomatic), but in some cases it may produce a feeling of pelvic pressure or heaviness or the sense that something is falling out of your vagina. It may even feel like you're sitting on a small ball. Leakage of urine may result, as well as symptoms of frequency and urgency, or you may have difficulty having a bowel movement. Discomfort with sexual activity also may develop.

Pelvic organ prolapse occurs because of a lack of pelvic floor muscle support. This can be the result of childbirth, as mentioned above, or estrogen deficiency associated with menopause. Other causes include congenital defects — problems that you were born with, such as a congenitally short vagina — and pelvic surgery, such as a hysterectomy or even a bladder suspension procedure that was done to treat incontinence. Chronic constipation, heavy lifting and chronic coughing also may contribute to prolapsed pelvic organs.

If you have pelvic organ prolapse but aren't experiencing any symptoms, treatment may not be necessary. In fact, treatment of asymptomatic prolapse may lead to new urinary, bowel or sexual problems. But if the condition is bothersome, your doctor may recommend conservative treatment at first, such as pelvic floor exercises, vaginal estrogen cream, the use of a pessary (for more on pessaries, see page 74) to provide additional pelvic support, and avoiding heavy lifting and straining. These treatments can also be used to address associated incontinence.

In cases of severe prolapse, surgery to restore normal positioning of the prolapsed organ may be an option. If incontinence is also present, surgery to treat both of these conditions may be done. (Chapter 6 has details on surgical procedures to treat incontinence.)

Menopause
The hormone estrogen plays a key role in regulating a number of important body functions in women. Among them, estrogen helps keep the tissues lining the vagina and urethra healthy and smooth. After menopause a woman's body produces less estrogen. As estrogen levels decline, vaginal and urethral tissues tend to become drier, thinner and less elastic. This affects their ability to close, meaning that one part of the protective mechanism that keeps a woman dry may be weakened. In addition, age-associated changes unrelated to hormonal changes can lead to a decrease in the bladder's storage capacity.

Some women experience a decline in estrogen production more rapidly than do others. When combined with weak pelvic muscle support and damage to the perineum resulting from childbirth or perhaps previous pelvic surgery, estrogen-deficient vaginal and urethral tissues can contribute to urinary incontinence. Some studies have found, however, that menopause in and of itself doesn't represent a strong risk of urinary incontinence.

If you experience urinary incontinence and it seems to be associated with hormonal changes due to menopause, your doctor may recommend estrogen therapy in the form of a vaginal cream, tablet or estrogen ring. Although there's no clear evidence that estrogen therapy improves incontinence, it can help tone and revitalize your vaginal and urethral tissues, which in turn may help prevent leakage of urine. (See Chapter 5 for more information on estrogen therapy.)

Pelvic surgery

In women, the bladder and uterus lie close to each other and are supported by the same pelvic floor muscles and ligaments. Any surgery that involves the reproductive system, such as removal of the uterus (hysterectomy), runs the risk of damaging muscles or nerves of the urinary tract, which can lead to incontinence.

Hysterectomy is one of the most common surgical procedures performed in women, second only to Caesarean section. Hysterectomy can be an effective treatment for many conditions, including gynecologic cancer, benign uterine tumors (fibroids), endometriosis, uterine prolapse and chronic vaginal bleeding.

Is urinary incontinence inevitable?

Certainly not. Not every woman who has had children develops incontinence and, in fact, some women who have never had children have incontinence problems. And in some women, hormones don't fluctuate as much as they do in other women during menopause.

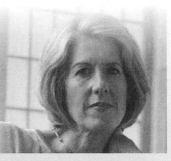

As women become more educated about incontinence, they can take preventive measures early in life to exercise and strengthen the muscles that support their reproductive and urinary systems (pelvic floor muscles). This will help reduce the physical stress wrought by different life stages and keep these muscles healthy and functional.

Although the risk of organ and tissue damage during a hysterectomy is certainly possible, studies of the relationship between hysterectomy and urinary incontinence have been inconclusive. If you're considering a hysterectomy, your doctor can help you assess its risks and benefits in your case.

Urogenital fistula

On rare occasions, an abnormal opening (fistula) between a part of your urinary tract — such as the bladder, urethra or ureter — and your vagina can lead to chronic, continuous urinary leakage. In developed countries, urogenital fistulas usually occur after pelvic surgery such as hysterectomy or bladder surgery. The fistula may be caused by injury during surgery, which typically results in immediate leakage, or later complications such as scar tissue or partial obstruction. In some cases radiation therapy can cause a fistula. In developing countries, urogenital fistulas are more often caused by complicated labor and delivery.

If an injury occurs and is noticed while surgery is taking place, your surgeon can repair it immediately. If you develop continuous leakage of urine after surgery and your doctor determines that it's caused by a fistula, additional surgery can be done to repair the opening.

Interstitial cystitis

Interstitial cystitis (IC) is a chronic inflammation of the bladder wall. It occurs primarily in women, and its signs and symptoms resemble those of a urinary tract infection. However, urine cultures of people with IC usually prove to be free of bacteria. Signs and symptoms include a frequent — sometimes urgent — need to urinate and chronic pelvic pain that may range from a mild burning sensation to severe pain.

No simple treatment exists to eliminate the signs and symptoms of IC, and no single treatment works for everyone. You may need to try various treatments or combinations of treatments before you and your doctor find the approach that relieves your signs and symptoms. Treatments include medications, nerve stimulation, bladder distention and surgery.

Men

In men urinary urgency, frequency and incontinence may be related to problems with the prostate gland. The prostate gland is part of the male reproductive system. About the size and shape of a walnut, it's located behind the pubic bone and in front of the rectum. The prostate's main function is to produce most of the fluids in semen, the fluid that transports sperm. Because of its location, it's also important to your urinary health. The prostate surrounds the neck of the bladder like a doughnut. When your prostate is healthy, this doesn't pose any problems. But if disease develops in the prostate, tissue in this gland can swell or grow, squeezing the urethra and affecting your ability to urinate. In addition, urinary incontinence may develop as a complication of surgery used to treat some of these problems.

Prostate problems aren't the reason behind all male urinary problems, including incontinence. For example, men may develop incontinence associated with urethral narrowing (urethral stricture). And, just as in women, incontinence may develop due to nerve damage, age-related changes or reasons that aren't known. Because treatment may vary for the different underlying problems, it's important to receive a thorough examination and assessment of your condition from your doctor so that you can pursue appropriate therapy.

Prostate disease

Three types of disease can affect the prostate gland: inflammation (prostatitis), noncancerous enlargement (benign prostatic hyperplasia, or BPH), and cancer. Of these three, BPH is the most common cause of urinary problems, including incontinence. But all three share signs and symptoms of overactive bladder and overflow incontinence, including:

- Difficulty starting your urine stream
- A weak urine stream
- Urinating more frequently, especially at night
- An urgent need to urinate
- Pain or a burning sensation while urinating

- Feeling as if your bladder isn't empty, even after you've just finished urinating
- Dribbling after you've finished urinating

It's important to note that prostate cancer produces few if any signs and symptoms in its early stages, which is why it's important to have regular prostate checkups to catch the disease early.

Prostatitis. Inflammation of the prostate gland can be caused by a bacterial infection or by another factor that's irritating the gland. If bacteria are the cause, antibiotics to treat the infection will generally resolve the frequency and urgency of urination associated with it.

Nonbacterial prostatitis is far more common than bacterial prostatitis but more difficult to diagnose and treat because its cause is unknown. As a result, treatment is often aimed at relieving symptoms. Your doctor may recommend the use of alpha blockers (see Chapter 5) to relax the muscles in your bladder neck and urethra and improve urine flow. Pain relievers, such as acetaminophen, aspirin or other nonsteroidal anti-inflammatory drugs (NSAIDs) can ease pain and discomfort. Other possible forms of treatment include physical therapy, which involves exercises to stretch and relax the lower pelvic muscles, and biofeedback (see Chapter 4). Soaking in warm water (a sitz bath) also may help.

If you have a bacterial form of the disease and antibiotics don't improve your symptoms or your fertility is severely affected, surgical treatment to open ducts blocked by inflammation may be used, though this is rare. Surgery isn't recommended for chronic nonbacterial prostatitis.

Benign prostatic hyperplasia. At birth your prostate gland is about the size of a pea. It grows slightly during childhood and then undergoes rapid growth during puberty. By age 25 your prostate is fully developed. Most men, however, experience a second period of prostate growth in their mid-40s. Frequently at this age, cells in the central portion of the gland — where the prostate surrounds the urethra — begin to expand more rapidly than normal. More than half of men in their 60s and up to 90 percent of those in their 70s and 80s have some symptoms of benign prostatic hyperplasia (BPH).

As tissues in the area enlarge, they often press on the urethra and obstruct urine flow. In addition, the bladder needs to work harder,

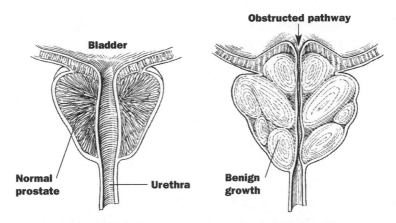

In men, the urethra, the tube that drains the bladder, is surrounded by the prostate gland. Benign prostatic hyperplasia (BPH) results when tissues in the central portion of the prostate gland enlarge and press on the urethra, affecting normal urine flow.

and its wall becomes thicker and more irritable. This can lead to increased bladder contractions, even when the bladder contains only small amounts of urine, and increased frequency of urination.

Why the prostate gland enlarges later in life is unclear. Researchers believe that with age the prostate may become more sensitive to the cell growth caused by male hormones such as testosterone. Fortunately, the condition varies in severity and it doesn't always pose a problem. Only about half the men with BPH experience signs and symptoms that are noticeable or bothersome enough to prompt medical treatment. A serious health threat arises when the condition prevents you from emptying your bladder normally. A bladder that's continually full can lead to recurrent bladder infection and sometimes to kidney damage.

Treatment. Treatment for BPH depends on the severity of your signs and symptoms. If your prostate is enlarged but you show no evidence of cancer and are experiencing little or no discomfort, treatment usually isn't necessary. If you have significant problems, a wide variety of treatments are available. In general, treatments aimed at easing signs and symptoms of BPH will also address those associated with urinary problems, including incontinence.

Medications are the first line of treatment and the most common method for controlling moderate symptoms of an enlarged prostate. These may include alpha blockers — such as terazosin

(Hytrin), doxazosin (Cardura) and tamsulosin (Flomax) — to relax muscles and improve urine flow (see Chapter 5) or finasteride (Proscar). Finasteride works by shrinking your prostate gland and is especially helpful for men with large prostates. It's not as effective for men with moderately enlarged or normal-sized prostates or for men with bladders that don't empty completely.

Your doctor may recommend taking doxazosin and finasteride together. Researchers found that this combination of drugs significantly reduced the risk of further prostate gland enlargement to the point where invasive surgery was not needed. This therapy also appears to decrease urination problems associated with BPH.

Medications aren't very effective in treating some types of prostate enlargement. Your urologist can advise you on what medication may be best in your case.

Another nonsurgical therapy for BPH includes use of prostatic stents. A prostatic stent is a tiny metal coil that's inserted into the urethra to widen it and keep it open. Stents aren't for everyone, as they may cause irritation when urinating or lead to frequent urinary tract infections. They can also be costly and potentially difficult to remove, which makes them a less popular alternative.

A number of surgical procedures — many of which are minimally invasive — are available for treating BPH. These are used mainly for treating severe signs and symptoms, or if you have complications such as frequent urinary tract infections, kidney damage, bleeding through the urethra or bladder stones. These procedures are very effective for relieving symptoms of BPH. The most common surgical technique is called transurethral resection of the prostate (TURP), where a surgeon threads a narrow instrument (resectoscope) into the urethra and uses small cutting tools to scrape away excess prostate tissue (see image on page 28).

A variation of this procedure, transurethral incision of the prostate (TUIP), may be helpful if your prostate has undergone changes that have led to a narrowing of the bladder neck. Instead of removing prostate tissue, the surgeon makes one or two cuts in the prostate gland to help enlarge the opening of the bladder neck.

Heat therapies — also called thermal therapies — are less invasive treatments than are TURP and TUIP. Heat therapies use various types of energy — including microwave, radiofrequency and laser — to create heat that destroys excessive prostate tissue.

Newer, high-energy lasers are also being used to destroy excess prostate tissue, either by cutting it out or by vaporizing it. The goal is to combine the advantages of laser therapy — safety and limited bleeding — with immediate improvement in urinary flow that usually comes with more invasive surgery.

Prostate cancer. A cancerous tumor in the prostate gland can press against or block the urethra and cause urination problems, such as overflow incontinence and urinary retention. But in its early stages, it usually doesn't cause any signs or symptoms. Because of this most doctors recommend that men begin prostate cancer screening at age 50 or earlier if you're at high risk. If you're black or have a family history of the disease — known risk factors for prostate cancer — you may want to begin screening at age 45.

Urinary incontinence is more often associated with the treatment for prostate cancer rather than the disease itself.

Treatment. Early-stage prostate cancer can be cured with two methods — surgery or radiation therapy. Surgical removal of your prostate gland (radical prostatectomy) is used to treat prostate cancer that hasn't spread outside of the gland. During the operation — done through an incision in your abdomen — your surgeon removes your entire prostate and the surrounding tissues and lymph nodes.

Radiation therapy also can be an effective way to treat prostate cancer. Radiation may be administered from a machine outside your body (external beam radiation) or through small radioactive pellets (seeds) implanted in your prostate gland (brachytherapy). Sometimes, both methods are used.

One of the potential complications of prostate cancer treatment is urinary incontinence. The nerves and muscles that help control urination lie close to the prostate gland and, depending on the size of the tumor and treatment technique used, it's possible that these nerves and muscles may be damaged during treatment. About 60 percent of men appear to have some degree of incontinence after surgery. In a national survey of Medicare recipients who underwent radical prostatectomy from 1988 to 1990, 30 percent reported needing to use incontinence products such as pads or clamps after surgery.

Among those who receive external beam radiation therapy, long-term urinary problems occur in fewer than 5 percent of men. The American Cancer Society reports that about one-third of men treated with brachytherapy develop increased urinary frequency.

For most men urinary incontinence after treatment is temporary. Normal bladder control gradually returns over several weeks or months as your tissues and nerves heal and strengthen. But for some, incontinence may become chronic. If you experience urinary incontinence after prostate cancer treatment, don't accept it as simply a price you have to pay for having cancer treatment. In many cases this problem can be successfully treated, so be sure to talk to your doctor about it.

One type of incontinence experienced after prostate cancer treatment is stress incontinence, resulting from a weakened sphincter muscle. This can result in leakage when physical activity puts extra pressure on your abdomen. To counteract this weakness, your doctor may suggest pelvic floor muscle training (see "Pelvic floor exercises" on page 191 of the Appendix). Biofeedback or electrical stimulation may also be used to treat stress incontinence (see Chapters 4 and 5 for more on these methods).

Incontinence may also occur because nerves that control storage of urine in the bladder have been damaged. This requires other types of treatment, often with the same medications used to treat overactive bladder.

Children

After birth it generally takes several years for a child to develop the skills needed to remain continent. Initially, a baby's bladder fills to a set-point, then contracts and empties automatically. As a child grows, the central nervous system matures and communication between the brain and bladder becomes more defined and efficient. Eventually, a child learns to urinate at will rather than as an involuntary reflex.

Still, accidents can and do often happen, particularly at night. This is not uncommon, and bladder control often improves with time. In fact, the rate of incontinence in children decreases by approximately 15 percent for each year after the age of 5. Wetting at night is called nocturnal enuresis. Diurnal incontinence is a term used for daytime wetting.

Delayed growth is the most common cause for incontinence in children, especially in those who have never been consistently dry. If your child develops incontinence after having been dry for a period of time, it may be due to a recurring urinary tract infection, an overactive bladder, inappropriate urinating habits or as a reaction to a stressful life event, such as the birth of a sibling or the first week of school. Less commonly, incontinence in children may be caused by a neurological condition or anatomical abnormality that's present at birth (a congenital condition).

Nighttime wetting

Nighttime wetting (nocturnal enuresis) is involuntary urination at night in a child age 5 or older. If your child has never been totally dry, this is known as primary enuresis. If your child was fully trained and then starts bed-wetting after a period of being completely dry, this is referred to as secondary enuresis.

Primary enuresis. Experts don't know the exact cause of primary enuresis, but it most likely arises from a mix of factors that include the following:

Small bladder capacity. Your child's bladder may not be developed enough yet to hold urine through the night.

Excessive nighttime production of urine. Up to adolescence, your child's body produces increased levels of an anti-diuretic hormone (ADH) at night. This causes urine production to slow and allows your child to sleep through the night without being bothered by a full bladder. But if your child's body isn't producing enough ADH at night, his or her bladder may fill to the point of overflowing.

Overactive bladder at night. Some children experience uninhibited bladder contractions at night, leading to bed-wetting. An overactive bladder at night usually is connected to daytime symptoms, such as frequency, urgency, "holding on" and low bladder capacity. If your child is having both daytime and nighttime signs and symptoms, he or she has functional incontinence. This is generally treated differently from nocturnal enuresis.

Inability to wake up or to make it to the toilet. Whether your child has a small bladder, excessive nighttime production of urine or an overactive bladder, bed-wetting occurs because of an inability to wake up to go to the toilet or practical difficulties in reaching the toilet when the bladder is full. Although children who bed-wet sleep normally — that is, they don't necessarily sleep any more deeply than other children — they're unable to rouse themselves when their bladders are full. Studies show that bed-wetting typically occurs in the first third of the night, which also happens to be when it's most difficult for all children to wake up. In some cases a child may wake up but may not want to get out of bed for fear of the dark or because it's cold. In these situations practical measures such as leaving a hall light on or keeping the room warm may help.

Genetics. Bed-wetting appears to run in families. If both parents experienced nocturnal enuresis as children, the chance of their children experiencing it is more than 70 percent.

When deciding on a treatment plan for your child, it's important to include your child in the discussion. Evidence indicates that when a child understands the emotional as well as the practical benefits of being dry and is motivated to stop wetting, treatment is generally more successful. In fact, in some cases, formal treatment may not even be necessary — about 20 percent of children become dry in the next eight weeks without any further treatment. Key ingredients to a positive treatment plan include:

- Instituting regular patterns of sleeping, eating and drinking throughout the day
- Limiting fluids before bedtime
- Keeping bedtime routines relaxed
- Stressing that the condition is common, isn't usually a sign of a psychological problem and often stops on its own

Additional methods for treating nocturnal enuresis include enuresis alarms, behavior therapy and medications. In general, researchers have found the alarm to be the most successful treatment for enuresis, although it's often combined with various behavior modification techniques or medications.

Enuresis alarm. An enuresis alarm is a device that attaches to your child's pajamas. When the pad starts to get wet, the alarm goes off, waking your child up. Upon waking, pelvic floor muscles tighten and stop the flow of urine, allowing your child to make his or her way to the toilet to finish urinating. The purpose of the alarm is to allow your child to learn to respond to the sensation of a full bladder. Alarms usually work best for children over age 7 who can eventually take some responsibility for waking and going to the toilet on their own. It generally takes about six to eight weeks for this type of therapy to be effective.

Behavior therapy. Behavior modification techniques may be helpful in encouraging your child to develop habits and behaviors that contribute to dryness, such as using the toilet regularly during the day, urinating before going to bed, or waking up to go to the toilet. You may want to create a reward system, such as a star chart or tokens for favorite activities, to encourage progress and cooperation with bedtime routines. Because bed-wetting itself is involuntary, avoid punishment and be sure to reward only those behaviors that are under your child's control. Other behavior techniques include scheduled toilet trips throughout the night that are gradually decreased as dryness increases.

Medications. Your doctor may recommend a medication called desmopressin (DDAVP) to increase ADH levels at night and reduce urine production. This medication is approved for use in children. Imipramine (Tofranil) is an antidepressant that may be used to treat nocturnal enuresis. (For more information on these medications, see Chapter 5.) Medications can provide short-term relief of symptoms, but they usually don't offer a cure.

Secondary enuresis. Secondary enuresis may develop temporarily as a result of anxiety due to stressful events, such as a family illness or separation from a parent. Tension in the family or negative attitudes regarding the wetting can exacerbate this anxiety, leading to more wetting and creating a cycle of wetting and anxiety. Behavior factors that may contribute to enuresis include difficulties in sleeping, eating or drinking patterns, lack of cooperation with parents, or self-esteem issues.

Some researchers argue that the rate at which a child first became dry influences his or her susceptibility to secondary enuresis when stress or a crisis arises.

If your child develops secondary enuresis, have him or her examined by a doctor to rule out any underlying physical problems, such as a urinary tract infection, seizure disorder or diabetes. If the problem appears to be a reaction to stress, then psychotherapy or family therapy may be helpful.

Diurnal incontinence

Diurnal incontinence is usually characterized by daytime wetting but may also include nighttime wetting. Diurnal incontinence is less common than nocturnal enuresis but similar to enuresis in that it often goes away on its own. If your child has more than the occasional accident during the day, a visit to your doctor is a good idea to find out what may be causing the incontinence. Diurnal incontinence is generally divided into the following categories:

Overactive bladder. As in adults, overactive bladder in children is characterized by an urgent need to urinate. Children, however, tend to counter this urge by voluntarily contracting their pelvic muscles in order to postpone a trip to the bathroom and minimize leakage. These signs and symptoms may become worse toward the end of the day, as fatigue and loss of concentration increases.

Delaying urination for extended periods of time can increase the risk of urinary tract infection. In turn, an infection can irritate the bladder and produce further symptoms of urgency and frequency. Damp clothing is also ideal for bacterial growth, which can lead to more infection. All of these factors combined can create a cycle of incontinence and recurrent infection that can sometimes be difficult to treat. Postponing trips to the bathroom to urinate can also lead to postponement of defecation, resulting in constipation and sometimes fecal incontinence.

Treatment for overactive bladder may include anticholinergic medications to decrease involuntary bladder muscle contractions, reduce the strength of the contractions and increase bladder storage capacity. Medical care may also include bladder training and treatment of associated urinary tract infections and constipation. (For more on anticholinergic medications, see Chapter 5.)

Abnormal urinating habits. Some children will urinate only long enough to reduce the urge, leaving the toilet without completely emptying the bladder, a practice called interrupted voiding. In other children, urine flow is characterized by periodic bursts of pelvic floor contractions so that the flow takes on a staccato pattern. In both of these conditions, the child is unable to completely relax the pelvic floor muscles. This may occur as a result of constantly trying to counter the urge to urinate, or it may be a learned behavior.

These abnormal urinary habits (dysfunctional voiding) can result in residual urine being left in the bladder, which increases the risk of urinary tract infection. Constipation also may be associated with dysfunctional voiding.

The goal of treatment is to relax the pelvic floor muscles to achieve normal urine flow and complete emptying of the bladder. This can be done through behavioral training, encouraging children to relax their pelvic muscles when going to the bathroom, take their time and make sure their bladder is fully emptied. If overactive bladder is present, anticholinergic medications may be added. When possible, try to prevent urinary tract infections and constipation, and if they occur, treat them.

Lazy bladder syndrome. Lazy bladder syndrome is the opposite of overactive bladder. Instead of symptoms of urgency and frequency, children with lazy bladder syndrome feel little or no urge to urinate. When they do go to the bathroom, they must strain their abdominal muscles to expel urine because the bladder fails to contract normally.

Treatment for lazy bladder syndrome consists of using clean, intermittent catheterization to empty the bladder, combined with treatment for infections and constipation.

Giggle incontinence. Some children experience leakage when they laugh. Exactly why this happens isn't known. The condition can affect boys and girls and can last into the teenage and occasionally adult years. In general, however, this type of incontinence goes away on its own. The drug methylphenidate (Ritalin) has proven effective in treating giggle incontinence in some children.

Neuropathic bladder and anatomical abnormalities

Incontinence caused by a nerve-damaging disease is often referred to as neuropathic bladder. In children, the most common cause of neuropathic bladder is spina bifida. Babies born with spina bifida typically have an outpouching of membranes covering the spinal cord (myelomeningocele) that causes the loss of neurological control of the legs, bladder or bowel. About one in every 1,000 babies is born with spina bifida.

Surgery is performed soon after birth to minimize the risk of infection and preserve existing function of the spinal cord. Increasingly, this condition is being diagnosed and even treated before the baby is born (prenatally). The hope is that this early treatment will help prevent subsequent complications, including incontinence.

Children with cerebral palsy may experience incontinence, but this is more often due to lack of mobility than nerve injury.

Treatment for neuropathic bladder primarily consists of clean intermittent catheterization and medical therapy, including anticholinergics or alpha-adrenergic agonists. Together, these treatment methods can result in continence in 70 percent to 90 percent of children with this condition.

Anatomical abnormalities, such as defects of the urethra or ureters, are rare but may cause incontinence. These are generally corrected with surgery.

Older adults

As you age, a number of changes take place in your body that may make incontinence more likely to occur. These changes include:

- Decreased bladder capacity
- Less elastic bladder walls
- Increased urine retention after urination
- Weakened pelvic floor muscles, particularly in women
- Increasingly overactive bladder
- Enlarged prostate in men

But just because these changes take place doesn't mean incontinence will occur. Some older adults experience all of these changes yet are continent. Aging is not a direct cause of incontinence. Rather, it increases the *risk* of incontinence. This is important to note because many older people feel that incontinence is an inevitable part of aging and therefore nothing can be done about it. In fact, research indicates that fewer than half the older adults with incontinence seek help for it. But in most cases treatment that applies to incontinence in younger people also applies to the condition in older people.

Overactive bladder is the most common type of incontinence in older adults. In addition, many people experience frequent urges to urinate but have weak bladder contractions (detrusor hyperactivity with impaired contractility, or DHIC), which makes it difficult to empty the bladder completely. This can lead to urine retention and, in severe cases, overflow incontinence. Stress incontinence is common among older women. Mixed incontinence is also common among older women, and may involve stress incontinence and overactive bladder.

The primary difference in incontinence between young and older people is that in older adults, a number of other conditions may be present that increase the risk of incontinence. Some of these are reversible, such as infection or restricted mobility, and some are not, such as dementia (see Chapter 2 for more information on causes associated with incontinence).

Thus, if you're an older adult with incontinence, in planning your treatment, you and your doctor will need to take into account the factors related to development of the incontinence, such as mental skills, mobility, manual dexterity, medical issues including bowel habits, and motivation, in addition to actual urinary tract problems. This is because addressing some of these other risk factors first may help to manage or alleviate the incontinence. Indeed, in some people, early management of certain risk factors can prevent incontinence from developing.

Assessment and evaluation

A thorough assessment and evaluation is essential to diagnosing anyone with incontinence. But because so many different factors may contribute to incontinence in older adults, including factors

Nocturia

Many adults find that as they become older, they need to get up more often during the night to go to the bathroom. Although most people find it acceptable to get up once during the night to urinate, having to get up multiple times can lead to a chain of results including disrupted sleep, drowsiness during the day and an increased risk of falling. In some cases, nocturia can lead to incontinence and bed-wetting.

The main causes of nocturia are a decrease in the bladder's ability to hold urine, overproduction of urine or a combination of the two. A smaller bladder volume generally results from aging. Increased production of urine may result from medical conditions, such as diabetes, congestive heart failure or kidney disease. In addition, excessive intake of fluids later in the day, long-term use of water pills (diuretics), or changes in posture from day to night that can lead to the transfer of fluid from swollen feet or hands to the kidneys and subsequently to the bladder may also increase urine output. Reduced production of anti-diuretic hormone (ADH) at night also can lead to increased urine production.

Some people mistake insomnia or waking because of sleep apnea or snoring as a need to go to the bathroom. This can also

not directly related to the lower urinary tract, a complete physical examination and continence assessment are typically done, in addition to consideration of the following areas:
- Thinking and judgment skills (cognitive abilities)
- Ability to move around
- Environment, including access to a toilet
- Degree of independence in terms of daily living activities
- Level of support or care
- Potentially reversible contributors to incontinence
- Medications being taken, many of which can lead to or worsen incontinence

In frail or disabled older adults, other factors also need to be taken into account, such as how bothersome the condition is to the person with incontinence or to the caregiver, the person's level of lead to nocturia. Treating the sleep disorder often addresses the nocturia.

Simple measures may help relieve symptoms of nocturia, including the following:

- Restricting fluid intake, particularly alcohol and caffeine, in the late afternoon and evening, although not total daily fluid intake
- Wearing compression stockings to reduce swelling in your legs and feet
- Elevating your feet at the end of the day to reduce swelling and encourage urination before you go to bed
- Changing the time you take medications

If these efforts don't work, your doctor may prescribe a diuretic late in the afternoon to eliminate fluid retention. Some studies have investigated the use of desmopressin (DDAVP), which is primarily used for bed-wetting in children and for nocturia in older adults. Although the drug may be beneficial for some people, it can cause fluid retention, which can be dangerous in people with heart disease and high blood pressure.

motivation and ability to cooperate with treatment, and other co-existing medical conditions (comorbidities).

Treatment

Age, frailty or disability should not keep a person from receiving treatment for incontinence. In general, older adults are eligible for the same treatment that's available for younger people, with a few caveats.

Behavior therapy. Pelvic floor muscle training, biofeedback, electrical stimulation and bladder training can be effective forms of therapy for older adults who are fit, alert and motivated to take part in their own treatment. For those who have a disability, are frail or have a cognitive impairment, assisted voiding or prompted voiding — where a caregiver periodically reminds the person to

Incontinence care for impaired adults

Diseases that damage the nervous system, such as multiple sclerosis, Parkinson's disease and stroke, can have an effect on bladder control and lead to incontinence. Diseases that cause dementia, such as Alzheimer's, may lead to incontinence due to impaired functioning.

In the beginning stages of a chronic disease, many people can care for themselves with a limited amount of help. But as the disease progresses, a caregiver becomes necessary to assist with the activities of daily living. For someone who's had a stroke, caregiving may be needed immediately after the event. Caring for someone who has incontinence due to a neurological condition is a challenging task and often requires a creative approach. Here are some suggestions that may help:

- Be sure to have the incontinence evaluated by a doctor. It may be due to a reversible condition, such as an infection or a medication. Treating the underlying problem in this case usually improves the incontinence.
- Provide frequent reminders to use the toilet. Generally, a pattern of every one to two hours works well. You may need to bring the person to the bathroom and provide help with clothing and seating.

urinate — can help prevent accidents and manage incontinence. (For more on behavior therapy, see Chapter 4.)

Medications. Incontinence medications are generally prescribed with caution for older adults because of the greater potential for side effects. Still, anticholinergics such as oxybutynin can improve the effectiveness of behavior therapy for overactive bladder and may be used in conjunction with bladder training or prompted voiding. In men with enlarged prostates, alpha blockers may be used to help empty the bladder.

But before medication is prescribed, it's a good idea to talk with your doctor about all the other medications you're taking to make sure they're not directly or indirectly contributing to incontinence. If so, your doctor may be able to adjust them to decrease the risk of

- Watch for nonverbal signs, such as pacing or other signs of agitation, that indicate the person needs to use the toilet. He or she may not recognize the feeling of a full bladder or may lack the verbal skills to state this need.
- Avoid clothing with complicated fasteners, such as button-fly jeans. Elastic waistbands work well.
- Leave the door to the bathroom open and a light on to help the person easily locate the room, particularly at night. Some caregivers put reflective tape on the floor in the shape of arrows that point to the location of the bathroom.
- For a person with dementia, put a picture of a toilet and a sign that reads "Toilet" on the bathroom door. Avoid the word *restroom* or *bathroom*, which may be taken literally.
- Dehydration is fairly common in older adults. Don't decrease fluids unless the person is drinking more than eight to 10 glasses a day. Withholding fluids may actually increase incontinence by making urine more concentrated, which can irritate the bladder and cause increased frequency and urgency. However, you may want to discourage more than one beverage after dinner to decrease the occurrence of nighttime incontinence.

incontinence. New medications are usually started at a low dose and gradually increased as necessary to relieve symptoms and minimize side effects.

Medications may sometimes have undesired effects. For example, many people with detrusor hyperactivity with impaired contractility (DHIC) have an overactive bladder but also experience signs and symptoms of urine retention, which can lead to overflow incontinence. Anticholinergics may help relax an overactive bladder muscle but may cause incomplete emptying of the bladder and urine retention, thus making the overflow incontinence worse.

Because medications can have mixed effects, they're typically reserved as a secondary form of therapy, usually in combination with behavior therapy.

Surgery. Age in and of itself isn't a reason to avoid surgery. Healthy older adults generally respond well to surgery for incontinence and generally can be treated in the same way as younger people. However, there's a risk of postoperative complications common to any surgery in an older person, including dehydration, infection, delirium and falls.

Because of the complex nature of incontinence in older adults and the increased risks associated with surgery, doctors typically do a careful evaluation of the incontinence, including urodynamic testing, to make sure that any reversible causes can be addressed before the surgery. In addition, it may be worthwhile to go through a trial of conservative treatment first, followed by a re-evaluation of the need for surgery. (For more on surgery to treat incontinence, see Chapter 6.)

Don't neglect to seek help

If you're an older adult and are experiencing incontinence or you're caring for an older adult with incontinence, seek help for this condition. Your doctor can help you find appropriate treatment and help you sort through the various factors that may be contributing to incontinence. Addressing these issues can improve bladder control as well as the quality of life of both the person with incontinence and the caregiver.

In a survey of nursing home residents, respondents said they preferred interventions designed to help them manage or control urinary incontinence over interventions designed to reduce loneliness, improve sleep or increase physical functioning. Clearly, continence is important to every person's well-being and dignity and is a worthwhile goal.

Chapter 8

Coping with urinary incontinence

The good news about urinary incontinence is that treatment for this condition is becoming more and more effective. For years people have managed their incontinence by using absorbent pads, wearing dark clothing, carrying an extra set of clothes or simply opting out of social settings and staying at home. Although these methods may help you avoid embarrassment, they don't address the incontinence itself.

Today there are better ways to manage urinary incontinence. Behavior therapies, medications and surgical procedures can substantially reduce, if not eliminate, urinary leakage and help you regain control of your bladder. In addition, new treatments are continually being discovered. This is why it's important to talk with a doctor, particularly one who is prepared to help you find the best treatment for your situation. If you can find a treatment that works — and most people do — you'll greatly minimize the effect of incontinence on your life.

Still, you may need to cope with the effects of incontinence while waiting for surgery or for medications or behavior therapies to gain effectiveness. And in some cases, treatment may not provide a complete cure. In such cases, you can use a number of practical, self-care strategies to deal with incontinence, such as reducing risks, changing your environment and becoming more comfortable with yourself.

Reducing your risk of incontinence

Although some risk factors for incontinence are outside of your control, such as aging or a spinal cord injury, you do have control over other factors, such as lifestyle choices. Eating well, exercising regularly and not smoking are basic components of a healthy lifestyle. Making such practices a part of your daily life can do a lot to reduce your risk of incontinence as well as many other diseases and conditions, including cardiovascular disease, stroke, high blood pressure, diabetes and some types of cancer.

Eating well

What goes into your body has a definite effect on your health. Choosing healthy foods that nourish and strengthen your bones, muscles, organs and other tissues is vital to helping you feel your best and reduce your risk of illness. The following actions may be specifically helpful for incontinence:

Shed extra pounds. If you're overweight — your body mass index (BMI) is over 25 — losing excess pounds can help reduce the overall pressure on your bladder, pelvic floor muscles and associated nerves. Studies suggest that losing 5 percent to 10 percent of your body weight can help improve signs and symptoms of incontinence. (To determine your BMI, see the BMI chart on page 23.)

Of the many ways to lose weight, crash diets are usually the least effective in the long term. One way to eat well and lose weight is to focus on foods that are low in energy density. Energy density is a ratio of calories to volume of food. Fruits and vegetables have low energy density. You can eat large amounts of them and still consume fewer calories than if you had eaten a small amount of a rich dessert or fried food, which generally has high energy density.

By replacing high-energy-dense foods with low-energy-dense foods, you'll satisfy those hunger pangs while consuming fewer calories, which will help you lose weight.

Add fiber to your diet. Constipation is an important contributor to incontinence. Keeping your bowel movements soft and regular allows urine to flow freely and reduces the strain that's placed on your pelvic floor muscles. Eating foods that are high in fiber —

whole grains, legumes, fruits and vegetables — can help to relieve and prevent constipation.

Avoid dietary bladder irritants. Avoiding or reducing food and drink that you know irritate your bladder can help relieve some symptoms of incontinence. For example, if you know that drinking coffee throughout the day has a tendency to make you go to the bathroom more frequently, you might reduce your caffeine intake to one or two cups a day. For a list of potential bladder irritants in your diet, see pages 188-191 in the Appendix.

Maintain proper fluid intake. Drinking too much fluid can make you urinate more frequently. But not drinking enough can lead to a concentration of waste in your urine, which can irritate your bladder and cause symptoms of urgency and frequency. According to the Institute of Medicine's guideline for water intake, letting your thirst be your guide typically gives you an adequate amount of fluid, both from drinks and food. As you get older, however, thirst and your perception of thirst changes, and thirst may not be the best guide for the amount of fluid you need. If you're experiencing incontinence, try to drink between 48 and 60 ounces (approximately six to seven 8-ounce cups) of fluid daily. This doesn't have to be just water — you can get fluids from tea, juice, and other beverages and foods, such as fruits, vegetables and soups.

Exercising

Thirty minutes or more of physical activity on most days is all you need to improve your fitness and gain the benefits of regular exercise. Regular physical activity can help you:

Stay fit, lose weight. Being physically active helps to keep your muscles, including your pelvic floor muscles, strong and flexible, and it can help control your weight.

Reduce your risk of prostate enlargement. In men, walking two or three hours a week can reduce the risk of developing an enlarged prostate, which is one of the most common causes of male incontinence.

Preserve independence. In older adults regular exercise preserves bone mass and muscle tone, improves fitness and helps maintain independence. This can reduce the risk of incontinence that's caused by restricted mobility or difficulty in managing zippers and buttons (functional incontinence). By strengthening your muscles and bones, you can also improve your balance and coordination, reducing your risk of falls.

Fight depression. Physical activity can help you combat depression, which has been associated with incontinence, especially in middle-aged women. Exercise fights depression by helping to balance brain chemicals that may be out of sync. Exercise also stimulates the production of endorphins — brain chemicals that produce feelings of well-being.

Note: Women who experience urine leakage while exercising may consider wearing a support device such as a urethral insert or a pessary. These devices support the bladder neck and help prevent leakage. Some women even use supertampons or a diaphragm as support devices. (For more on medical devices used to treat incontinence, see Chapter 5.)

Not smoking
Smoking can lead to a severe chronic cough, which can aggravate the symptoms of stress incontinence. Stopping smoking can relieve your coughing and reduce the pressure that coughing places on your bladder and pelvic floor muscles.

Stopping smoking is often easier said than done, but it's not impossible. Furthermore, stopping smoking has many benefits in addition to improving symptoms of incontinence, including lowered risk of lung cancer, cardiovascular disease and infertility.

Stopping smoking generally involves using several strategies. Combining medications (Nicorette, NicoDerm CQ, Zyban) with follow-up visits to your doctor for support and counseling is usually more successful than trying to stop on your own. Smoking cessation programs also offer supportive guidance to stopping.

Changing your environment

If you have trouble getting to the bathroom on time because of restricted mobility, perhaps because of arthritis or recent hip surgery, modifying your personal environment may help you prevent incontinence episodes. Some changes that may be helpful include the following:

- Choosing a bedroom or sleeping area that's close to the bathroom
- Keeping the way to the bathroom well lighted and free of obstacles such as throw rugs, which may trip you and cause a fall
- Installing an elevated toilet seat (some have arm rests) so that it's easier to sit down and get up
- Installing grab bars to help you get on and off the toilet
- Keeping a bedpan or urinal in your bedroom
- Having a commode (portable toilet) nearby if your only bathroom is up or down a flight of stairs.

If you need more extensive changes, you might consider adding another bathroom to your house in a more convenient location or widening an existing bathroom doorway.

Consulting an occupational or physical therapist also may be helpful. Occupational therapists specialize in helping people deal with the effects of aging, illness or injury in the management of their daily lives. An occupational therapist can meet with you on an individual basis and make recommendations based on your needs.

In addition, using assistive devices such as canes and walkers can help you move around faster, more easily and more safely. Different types and sizes of walking aids are available. A physical therapist or your family doctor can help you find a cane or walker that fits you properly.

Minimize clothing difficulties

If you have an overactive bladder and you're just starting on a bladder-training program, it may help to decrease the number of articles of clothing you wear that might get in the way of toileting.

For example, women may choose to wear just a dress and a pair of underwear and eliminate pantyhose and slips for the time being. Men may choose to wear suspenders or pants with an elastic waistband instead of a belt. This way you won't be fumbling with clothing even as your sense of urgency increases. As you gain more control of your bladder through training or timed voiding, you can feel more comfortable wearing pantyhose or belts.

Going out and about

Try not to let incontinence keep you away from work or social settings outside your home. In fact, it's essential that you maintain your connection with family, friends and colleagues because this type of support network can prevent the feelings of isolation and depression that can accompany incontinence. Getting out of the house for lunch with a friend or for a movie with your spouse can refresh your perspective and give your spirits a boost.

Behavior therapies such as pelvic floor muscle training and bladder training can help you gain better control over your bladder so that you can last through a meeting at work or a movie at the theater without having to go to the restroom. In the meantime, however, being prepared may make you more comfortable when you're out and about. The following tips may be helpful. But remember, these are short-term methods for relieving the symptoms of incontinence. They aren't considered a primary form of treatment.

Stock up on supplies. When going out, take an adequate supply of incontinence pads or protective undergarments with you. This way, if leakage does occur, you can feel confident knowing you can replace a used product with a fresh one and not have to go home immediately. Today's products are becoming ever more discreet and can easily fit into a roomy purse or small backpack. You may also wish to carry a change of clothes with you. Even a sweater wrapped around your waist can come in handy in case of an emergency. You can use a zippered plastic bag to contain any soiled clothing until you get home.

People who travel a lot often keep a bag of toiletries at the ready so they don't need to repack it every time they leave. You could do the same, keeping a bag with all of your necessary supplies by the door, so you can simply grab it on your way out. You might even keep some extra supplies in your car in case you forget your bag.

If you're planning on being physically active, you might think about wearing a urethral insert or foam patch. These devices can prevent leakage during your planned activity and can be discarded later. (See Chapter 5 for more information on incontinence devices.)

Scout out your destination. Familiarize yourself with the restrooms available at the place you're going to. If you're at a movie theater or a religious service, you may wish to sit near the aisle so that you can easily get up and go to the restroom if necessary. If you're with an older adult who has a problem with incontinence, you might go to the restroom yourself every couple of hours and offer him or her the opportunity to go with you. This saves them the embarrassment of having to ask or be asked to go to the restroom.

Take good care of yourself. When leakages are addressed promptly, odor and skin irritation are rarely more than a momentary problem. If you're experiencing leakage, take good care of your skin and keep it as dry as possible. Prolonged contact with wet clothing can cause the skin to break down, resulting in irritation and sores. See "Self-care products for incontinence" on pages 126-127 for more information on products to help you stay clean and dry.

Sexuality and incontinence

Sexuality and incontinence are topics that many people find difficult to talk about, and combining the two into one conversation can be even harder. Certainly incontinence can have a negative effect on your sex life if you let it. But it doesn't necessarily have to get in the way of intimacy, and it may not have as much importance as you think.

Leaking urine during sexual intercourse can be upsetting. Women with stress incontinence may find that they leak urine at the beginning of intercourse when their partner's penis presses against the urethra and bladder upon initial penetration. In women with urge incontinence, urine leakage may be more unpredictable, though it often occurs during orgasm, and in greater volume than in women with stress incontinence. Urgency and frequency in both

Self-care products for incontinence

A wide variety of incontinence self-care products are available. Which ones you choose depend on the volume of urine you tend to lose, when you typically experience leakage, how easy a product is to use, and its cost, comfort, odor control and durability. Your doctor or nurse can help you choose products that will help you most.

You can find incontinence care products at drugstores or medical supply stores and through companies that sell durable medical equipment. The National Association For Continence (NAFC) offers to its members a supply catalog called *Resource Guide: Products and Services for Incontinence.* A one-year subscription costs $25 for consumers and includes a newsletter, a print version and online access to the *Resource Guide,* and a number of other publications and resources. You might also check with your doctor or therapist — he or she may have a copy of the catalogue that you can look at. You can visit the NAFC's Web site at *www.nafc.org* or call (800) BLADDER, or (800) 252-3337.

Here's a look at some categories of products available.

Bladder control pads

Disposable pads designed to manage urine leakage are similar to sanitary pads but are much more absorbent and have a waterproof backing. They are worn inside your underwear and discarded after use. Some have an elastic leg for a better fit. Absorbent products generally incorporate three layers: a top layer that wicks away moisture from your skin, a middle layer that absorbs the moisture and an outer layer that may be waterproof to keep the moisture in or breathable to allow the moisture to evaporate.

Sanitary pads and panty liners may work for very small amounts of leakage, but they generally aren't as absorbent as incontinence pads. For men, there are also absorbent pouches available that fit inside your briefs.

Protective undergarments

Protective undergarments are often worn in place of your normal underwear. Different types available include:

Pull-ons. Pull-ons function exactly as the name suggests. You pull them up over your legs and wear them like traditional underwear. They're available in either disposable or reusable forms. The disposable forms (Attends Pull-Ons, Depend Protective Underwear, SureCare Slip-On Undergarment) come in a variety of sizes and absorbencies.

The reusable undergarments are washable and come in a couple of varieties. One is made of waterproof material and is designed to be worn as an extra layer of protection over absorbent pads or undergarments (Sani-Pant Pull-On Brief). The other kind is newer and is designed to absorb and protect just like a disposable, but it can be washed and reused (Salk's HealthDri).

Adult briefs. These products attach around your hips with either refastenable tape tabs (Attends Confidence, Depend Fitted Brief, Kendall Adult Brief, Attends Classic, Whitestone UltraShield, Wings) or reusable belts (Attends Belted Undergarment, Depend Belted Undergarment, Kendall Belted Undergarment). They're useful for containing large amounts of urine. Some are designed especially for overnight use. Adult briefs are available in both disposable and reusable forms and come in a variety of sizes. Some are contoured to better fit the outline of your body.

Skin care and odor products

Disposable cleansing wipes (Wings, Comfort Shield) and cleansing sprays or foams (Aloe Vesta, Prevacare, Baza, Bedside Care, Baby Comfort) are gentler to your skin than toilet paper, moisturize and help eliminate odor. Baby wipes work well, too.

Special creams, gels or ointments (Aloe Vesta, Proshield) can be used to create a barrier against moisture and keep your skin dry. Some ointments (Calmoseptine) also work to heal irritated skin while acting as a moisture barrier.

Some people sprinkle a powder, such as baking soda or a vaginal powder, over a pad or garment to help absorb odor. Room sprays also help neutralize odor (Medi-Aire Bio, Odor Eliminator). Some products can be used on your skin and with your laundry (Mentor Skin and Appliance Odor Eliminator).

men and women may prevent you from feeling relaxed during a sexual experience.

Men who have incontinence associated with prostate cancer treatment may also have erectile dysfunction, a common side effect of prostate surgery. In this case, erectile dysfunction is likely to be a greater factor in sexual discomfort than is incontinence. Men don't usually leak urine during intercourse because of penile engorgement.

A 2002 study of more than 300 women over the age of 45 with urinary incontinence or advanced pelvic organ prolapse found that about one-fifth of the women cited their condition as a reason for sexual inactivity. Prolapse was a more common reason than urinary incontinence, and overactive bladder more common than stress or mixed incontinence. Among the women who were in an intimate relationship and sexually active, however, overall sexual satisfaction was relatively unaffected by their condition or by treatment. A questionnaire sent out to the participants who were sexually active revealed that in the majority of women — regardless of whether they had prolapse, stress incontinence, overactive bladder or mixed incontinence — urine leakage or prolapse had no effect on their ability to have sexual relations.

The authors of the study recognized that sexual satisfaction depended on complex interactions and that physical health was only one of many contributing factors. Others included physiology, emotions, experiences, beliefs, lifestyle and a person's relationship with his or her partner. The study cited above suggested that incontinence may not be as great a detriment to sexual activity as is commonly thought.

If you feel that problems with incontinence are affecting your sex life or your sexuality in general — how you feel about yourself as a sexual being — consider having a frank discussion with your doctor or therapist. Although this type of conversation may seem too embarrassing to initiate at first, it can bring positive results in the form of treatment and management of your incontinence. Successful management of your incontinence can increase your confidence in yourself and your ability for sexual expression.

In the meantime, the following suggestions may help improve your sex life.

Talk with each other. As difficult as it may seem initially, talk with your partner about your condition. Obviously, it's important to have a loving partner to begin with, but you may be surprised at how understanding and willing to accommodate your partner can be. In any intimate relationship, regardless of how young or healthy the couple, open communication is probably the most important element in achieving mutual satisfaction. If necessary, seek professional help in breaking down communication barriers between you and your partner.

Expand your definition of sex. There are countless variations on sexual intimacy. Touch can be a good alternative to intercourse. It can simply mean holding each other. It can also mean sensual massage, mutual masturbation or oral sex.

Try a different position. Maybe a different position makes intercourse easier for you. If you're in a comfortable position, you're more likely to feel free to concentrate on making love and may be less prone to leakage. If you're a woman, being on top generally gives you better control of your pelvic muscles. Rear entry may ease pressure on your bladder. Ask your partner about his or her needs and ways that you can also be accommodating.

Empty your bladder beforehand. To reduce your chances of leakage during lovemaking, avoid drinking fluids for an hour or so before sex and empty your bladder immediately before starting.

If you're a woman, wear a diaphragm. Because of where a diaphragm sits in a woman's pelvic area, it can provide support to the bladder and urethra and help prevent leakage.

Do your Kegels. Pelvic floor muscle exercises (Kegels) can help strengthen your pelvic floor muscles and reduce leakage. In women, stronger pelvic muscles may lead to increased lubrication during foreplay and intercourse, enhanced vaginal sensation and orgasmic response, and a greater ability to respond to your partner, making sex more satisfying for both of you.

Be prepared. Having towels handy or using disposable pads on your bed may help ease some of your anxiety if you're worried about wetness.

Keep a sense of humor. Remember that sex is rarely as perfect as it appears in the movies. People are human, and if it's not one particular problem, it may be another. A sense of humor can help you overcome problems and even create greater intimacy between you and your partner.

Keeping a positive outlook

If incontinence has become a part of your life, you may find that it engenders emotions and behaviors that can be decidedly negative. A number of studies have found that depression is frequently associated with incontinence and that incontinence can have a negative effect on quality of life. If your incontinence is severe, you may begin to withdraw from social situations and isolate yourself from others, including your family, for fear of having an accident or that an odor may be present.

Whenever a part of you doesn't work as it used to or as it should, it's natural to feel a sense of loss, even if the change isn't exactly permanent. Toileting skills especially are acquired at a very young age and losing control of something that used to be second nature can trigger surprisingly intense feelings of grief, anger and despair. Some of the things you may miss include:

- Your sense of dignity
- Your independence
- Your privacy
- Spontaneity
- An enjoyable hobby or sport
- Sexual intimacy as it was before
- Untroubled family relationships
- Gatherings with friends
- Feelings of energy and confidence
- A sense of happiness and control over your life
- Job satisfaction

These are difficult losses. You may feel as if you're losing the things that give your life meaning and purpose. Your natural response is to grieve. Feelings that are often associated with grief include denial of the problem, anger, frustration, depression, guilt and shame.

Part 2

Fecal incontinence

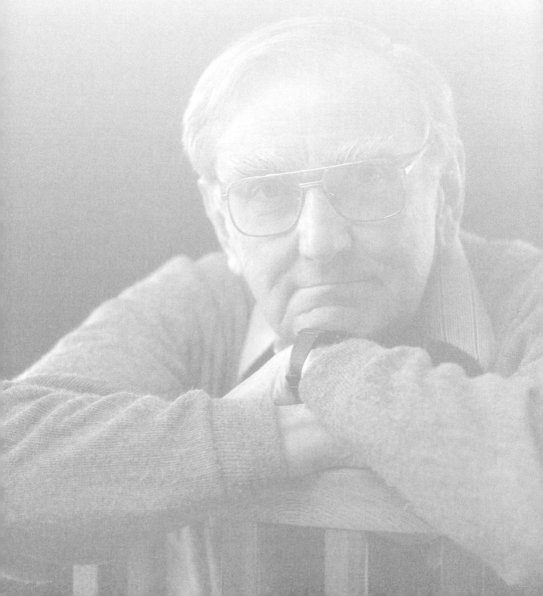

Chapter 9

Your bowels and incontinence

Fecal incontinence is not something you hear much about, although it affects more than 6 million Americans. Fecal incontinence is the inability to control your bowels. When you need to have a bowel movement, you may not be able to hold it long enough to reach a bathroom. This is called urge fecal incontinence. Or you may experience unexpected leakage of stool when you don't feel any urge to go. This is known as unsensed fecal incontinence.

Most of us take it for granted that we can control our bowels. We generally don't have an "accident" unless we have a short-lived bout of diarrhea. But that's not the case for people with chronic (recurring) fecal incontinence. They can't control the passage of gas or stool, which may be liquid or solid.

Fecal incontinence can range from occasional minor leakage to a complete loss of control of bowel movements. People with fecal incontinence may also pass gas involuntarily. Although the involuntary passing of gas in itself isn't defined as fecal incontinence, it can be a distressing problem.

Many people with urinary incontinence also have fecal incontinence — this is referred to as double incontinence. For example, an estimated 30 percent of women with urinary incontinence have also had episodes of fecal incontinence.

Fecal incontinence can have a devastating effect on nearly every aspect of your daily life, including your self-image, your work and your relationships. As you try to manage a bodily process that can't be controlled, your confidence, self-respect and composure can falter. You may feel ashamed, embarrassed or humiliated.

Many people with fecal incontinence are afraid to leave the house in case they have an accident in public. They feel as if they're "tethered to the toilet." It can be hard to take a walk around the block, let alone ride in a car, bus or airplane. Social functions are daunting, to say the least. Keeping a job can be challenging.

Most people with fecal incontinence don't tell anyone about it, not even their doctors. Instead, they limit their activities and withdraw from friends and family. The results can be social isolation, job loss, lowered self-esteem, depression and anxiety. In older adults, fecal incontinence is one of the most common reasons for nursing home placement.

Fecal incontinence is more common in older people, but it can affect anyone, including children after they've been toilet trained. It's difficult to determine how common the problem is, since many people are reluctant to report it. But an estimated 2 percent to 7 percent of the general population and 11 percent of people age 80 and older are affected. Among nursing home residents, the prevalence rises to about 45 percent. Women are more likely than are men to tell their doctors that they have fecal incontinence. But it's common among men as well as women.

Bowel warning signs

If fecal incontinence includes bleeding, see your doctor promptly. Bleeding, along with a lack of bowel control, may indicate inflammation of the colon (colitis), a rectal tumor or descent of the rectum into the anal canal (rectal prolapse). Other medical conditions, such as hemorrhoids, an anal injury or a rupture in the rectum (fistula), may allow mucus or blood to leak out through the anus. This leakage sometimes can be mistaken for fecal incontinence.

Even though fecal incontinence often affects older people, it's not a normal part of aging. And it's not a hopeless situation, no matter what your age. Improvements in the understanding, awareness, diagnosis and treatment of the problem have brightened the outlook for people with fecal incontinence. Most people can be helped with proper treatment, and often the problem can be resolved completely.

Taking steps to deal with fecal incontinence will help ease the embarrassment, fear, anxiety and loneliness that often come with the physical problems. Treatment can improve your life and help you feel better about yourself. This chapter will help you understand what causes fecal incontinence, how your bowels work and what happens if something goes wrong.

How your bowels work

Fecal incontinence isn't a specific disease. Rather, it's a sign of one or more medical problems. It can happen when something goes wrong with the complex, coordinated process that allows you to hold stool in until you choose to release it. Incontinence can result from a variety of problems and is rarely due to a single factor. To understand the causes of fecal incontinence, it's helpful to know something about the way your bowels normally work.

Continence is a function of a healthy digestive system. Your digestive tract begins at your mouth and ends at the rectum and anus in the lower portion of the large intestine. The digestive tract consists of several organs that work together to process the food you eat, absorb vital nutrients and fluids into the bloodstream, and remove waste that your body can't digest.

When your bowels are functioning normally, waste material progresses in an orderly fashion through the last part of the digestive tract — the large intestine (colon), rectum and anus. By the time food has slowly made its way through the lengthy digestive tract to the end of your colon, the nutrients have been absorbed. In the colon, nearly all of the water is removed from the waste. The remaining residue, called stool or feces, is usually soft but formed.

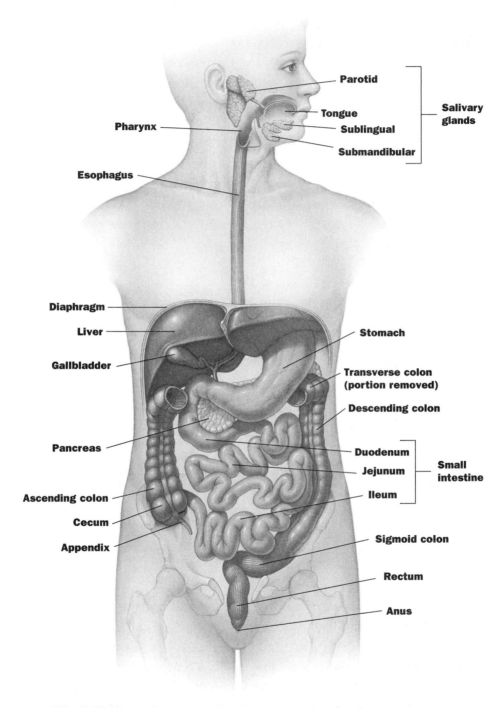

The digestive tract begins at the mouth and ends at the rectum and anus. It includes several vital organs.

Feces are made of undigested food, unabsorbed water, bacteria, mucus and dead cells. They're stored in the rectum before being released through the anus.

Bowel function is mainly controlled by three things:

- The strength of your anal sphincters, the ring-like muscles at the end of the rectum. These muscles tighten (contract) to prevent stool from leaving your rectum.
- The storage capacity of your rectum, allowing you to hold stool for some time after you're aware the stool is there.
- The ability to sense the need to pass stool.

To remain continent, your colon, rectum, anus and nervous system all have to be working normally. In addition, you have to be able to recognize and respond to the urge to go to the bathroom. Other factors that play a role include how food and waste move through your colon and the consistency and amount of stool.

Your colon

The colon, also called the large intestine or bowel, is about 5 feet long. It extends from the point where it joins the small intestine, in the lower right side of your abdomen, up toward the liver. From there it crosses the top of your abdomen, then turns sharply downward along the left side of the abdomen toward your pelvis. The last sections of the colon — the sigmoid colon, rectum and anus — are crucial to continence.

The lower part of the colon that descends from the top of the pelvic bone to the rectum is called the sigmoid colon. The name refers to its S-shaped curve (from the Greek word *sigma,* or *S*). The sigmoid colon helps to slow the passage of fecal material before it moves into the rectum.

It can take as long as 10 hours to several days for digestive contents to move through the entire colon. As it does, most of the fluid and salts are absorbed from the material. It dries out and becomes more solid, in the form of stool. Stool is stored in the sigmoid colon until muscle contractions move it into the rectum.

These muscle movements, known as peristaltic waves, rapidly propel stool forward toward the rectum. Peristaltic waves usually last for about 10 to 15 minutes two or three times a day, most

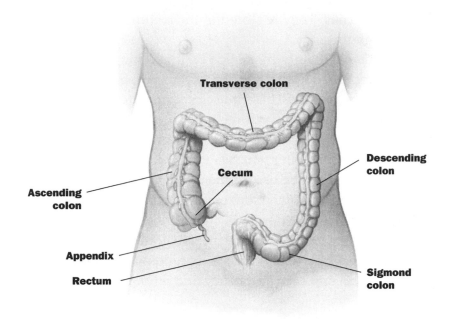

Your colon consists of four sections, beginning at the point where it joins the small intestine at the cecum and ending with the sigmoid section, just above the rectum.

commonly after awakening or after a meal. That's why many people grab the newspaper and head to the bathroom after breakfast. Eating also increases an activity of the colon called the gastrocolic reflex, which can make you feel like you need to use the bathroom.

Your rectum and anal canal

The rectum lies at the end of the large intestine, just after the sigmoid colon. The rectum is a hollow muscular tube about 5 inches long. It's more elastic than the rest of the bowel is, so it can expand to store fecal material. Normally the rectum is empty. When stool is pushed into the rectum from the colon, its walls stretch to accommodate it. The rectum is surrounded by nerves that sense the expansion and trigger the urge to have a bowel movement. As more stool enters the rectum, the urge increases.

As the rectal walls stretch, the internal anal sphincter muscle relaxes. The internal anal sphincter is one of two circular layers of muscle surrounding the last 2 inches of the rectum, called the anal canal. The anal canal ends at the anus — the opening at the end of the digestive tract. Most of the time, the internal anal sphincter stays tightened (contracted) to prevent leakage from the rectum into the anal canal.

But when the rectum expands, the internal anal sphincter opens briefly and lets a tiny bit of the rectum's contents come into contact with the many nerve endings in the anal canal. In a rapid "sampling reflex," sensory nerve receptors detect whether the rectal contents are gas or liquid or solid stool. This allows you to decide what to do — pass gas or hold it in, look for a bathroom quickly if you have diarrhea or loose stool, or wait for a more convenient time or place.

During this time, stool is held in, thanks to your external anal sphincter muscle. As your rectum expands, the external sphincter tightens. It's a unique muscle in that it can be tightened consciously, as when you constrict it to hold stool in, or by reflex (without conscious control). For example, when you're sleeping the internal and external anal sphincters stay contracted to keep stool from leaving the rectum. This reflex also kicks in when you cough, laugh

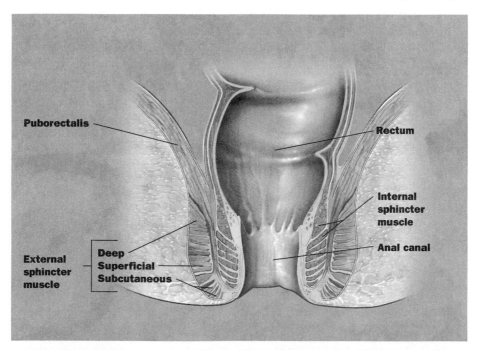

The external and internal anal sphincter muscles work together with the muscles of the rectum to control the passage of stool. When the anal sphincter muscles are damaged or weakened, fecal incontinence may result.

heartily or lift something heavy, so that the sudden increase in pressure in your abdomen doesn't force stool out.

Holding stool in

If you need to delay having a bowel movement, you tighten your external anal sphincter. You also contract a muscle called the puborectalis in your pelvic floor. This U-shaped muscle forms a sling that supports the area between the rectum and the anal canal. When the puborectalis muscle is contracted, it pulls the rectum so that it lies at an angle — above and to the side of the anal canal, rather than straight above it. This prevents feces from passing from the rectum into the anal canal.

You can actively tighten your external anal sphincter muscle for only a few minutes at the most. After that, your rectum stretches to hold more stool, the sense of urgency subsides and the external sphincter relaxes. The internal anal sphincter closes, keeping stool in the rectum.

The rectum's ability to stretch and store stool is known as compliance. Of course, there comes a point when the rectum is holding all the stool it can and you'll feel an urgent need to go to the bathroom. In most people, the rectum can comfortably hold up to about 300 milliliters of material (about 10 ounces, or a little over 1 cup). After that, things get decidedly uncomfortable.

Moving your bowels

When you're ready to have a bowel movement, all the muscles involved in maintaining continence — the internal and external anal sphincters and the puborectalis — relax. When you sit or squat, the angle between the anus and rectum straightens, allowing the contents of the rectum to move into the anus. As you push, your external anal sphincter and puborectalis muscles relax, further straightening the angle (see image on page 143).

To propel stool downward, you may bear down, a movement called the Valsalva maneuver. This closes off the airway, tightens the abdominal muscles and pushes the diaphragm down. The Valsalva maneuver increases pressure in your abdomen and helps empty the rectum.

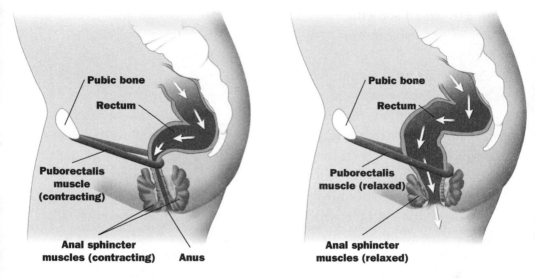

When the puborectalis muscle contracts (left), it holds the rectum at an angle such that stool is prevented from passing into the anal canal. As the puborectalis muscle relaxes (right), the angle is changed, allowing stool to move into the anal canal.

Bowel problems and incontinence

For your bowels to function normally and keep you from unintended bowel movements, all of the different, interconnected structures described in the preceding section have to be working together. Think of the digestive tract as something like a factory production line — members perform various functions at various sites to process food and fluids into an end result, feces. If any member of the line breaks down or stops working — in other words, if part of the system is affected by disease or injury — incontinence may result. Most often, more than one factor is involved.

Sometimes, incontinence occurs when an unrelated condition, such as arthritis, makes it physically difficult to reach the toilet when you need to go. This is referred to as functional incontinence.

Causes of fecal incontinence
Common causes of fecal incontinence include chronic (recurring) constipation, diarrhea, and muscle or nerve damage. Muscle damage is involved in most cases of fecal incontinence.

The muscles and nerves in and around the rectum and anus interact to sense the presence of waste, allow it to be stored, propel it along and, finally, eliminate it. Damage to the anal sphincter muscles can result in incontinence. The weakened muscles can't close tightly, so stool leaks out.

The pelvic floor muscles also play an important role in maintaining continence. These muscles support the organs within the pelvis and lower abdomen. If the pelvic floor muscles become weak or their function is disturbed, fecal incontinence can result.

Nerve damage can also play a role in fecal incontinence. To remain continent, a person must be able to recognize and respond to the urge to defecate. Conditions that affect your nervous system or cause nerve damage may decrease your awareness or sensation of bowel fullness. If the nerves that control the sphincter muscles are injured, they won't work properly and incontinence can occur. If the nerves that sense stool in the rectum are damaged, you may not feel the need to use the bathroom until stool has leaked out.

A broad range of conditions and disorders can cause fecal incontinence. These include:

Constipation. Chronic constipation stretches and weakens the anal sphincter muscles. This may make the nerves of the anus and rectum less responsive to the presence of stool in the rectum. In addition, constipation may weaken muscles of the colon. This slows down transit time in the bowel, making it difficult to pass stools and worsening the constipation.

Chronic constipation often leads to impacted stool, a large mass of hard, dry stool that becomes stuck in the rectum. Liquid stool then leaks out around it.

Diarrhea. Diarrhea, or loose stool, is more difficult to control than is formed, solid stool. Diarrhea can overwhelm your body's ability to hold stool in. Diarrhea may be due to many things, including infectious illnesses such as food poisoning or stomach flu, or overuse of laxatives. In addition, radiation therapy, certain medications, and diseases that affect the colon or rectum, such as ulcerative colitis, diverticular disease and cancer, can also cause diarrhea. Chronic diarrhea-causing conditions, such as inflammatory bowel disease (IBD) and irritable bowel syndrome (IBS), can result in incontinence.

Who's at risk?

Fecal incontinence can affect men and women, young people and old. Even people who don't have fecal incontinence may have an occasional "accident" when they have the stomach flu or other infectious disease that causes diarrhea.

Some factors increase your likelihood of incontinence, however. These risk factors include:

- Being unable to perform daily living activities, such as dressing yourself or going to the bathroom on your own
- Growing older
- Having chronic diarrhea or constipation
- Being in poor general health
- Giving birth, especially if you've had large babies, a long second stage of delivery, forceps deliveries, breech birth, a cut to extend the vaginal opening (episiotomy) or a vaginal tear that reached the anus
- Having colon, rectal, anal or gynecologic problems
- Taking certain medications
- In children, late or interrupted toilet training

In addition, diseases and conditions that increase your risk of fecal incontinence include:

- Diabetes
- Stroke
- Multiple sclerosis
- Parkinson's disease
- Systemic sclerosis
- Myotonic dystrophy
- Amyloidosis
- Spinal cord injuries
- Imperforate anus
- Hirschsprung's disease
- Genital and rectal prolapse (procidentia)

Irritable bowel syndrome. This disorder can cause loose stools and diarrhea, which are harder to control than are formed stools. (See "Irritable bowel syndrome and incontinence," on page 150.)

Neurological conditions. Multiple sclerosis, dementia, stroke, diabetes, spinal cord injuries and brain injuries can impair the ability to sense stool in the rectum.

Childbirth. Giving birth vaginally may cause weakness or damage in pelvic floor muscles and nerves. The risk of injury is greatest if you tear a muscle in your anus during delivery. Other factors that increase the likelihood of damage include the use of forceps during delivery, a large baby, a long second stage of delivery, a cut to enlarge the vaginal opening for delivery (episiotomy) and breech birth.

Incomplete emptying of rectum. Holding stool in the rectum for long periods or not emptying the rectum completely may lead to liquid stool seeping out.

Straining to defecate. A long-term habit of straining to go to the toilet can damage the nerves that sense stool in the rectum and can weaken the pelvic floor muscles.

Birth defects in anus or rectum. People born with problems affecting the anus or rectum may have lifelong issues with fecal incontinence.

Accidental injury. Injury to the pelvic floor, anus or rectum can damage muscles and nerves, causing incontinence.

Surgery. Surgery to treat enlarged veins in the rectum or anus (hemorrhoids) can damage the anus and cause fecal incontinence. Other operations involving your rectum and anus, as well as gynecologic, prostate and bowel surgeries, also may lead to fecal incontinence.

Medications. Medications that may cause or worsen fecal incontinence are listed in the Appendix on pages 194-195.

Scarring of rectum. It can be difficult to hold stool, particularly diarrhea, if the rectum walls lose elasticity, becoming stiffer and less able to stretch. This can occur as a result of scarring from rectal surgery, radiation treatment or IBD.

Other conditions. A dropping down of the rectum into the anus (rectal prolapse) or, in women, a protrusion of the rectum through

Aging and fecal incontinence

Fecal incontinence isn't an inevitable part of aging. For most people, bowel function remains vigorous and healthy well into old age. But some of the bodily changes that occur with aging can contribute to incontinence.

Over time, your anal sphincter muscles and the muscles and ligaments that support your pelvis can weaken. Older women are especially prone to lose strength in these areas, most likely because female reproductive hormones influence the strength and vigor of the pelvic floor and anal muscles. After menopause, when a woman's hormone levels drop sharply, the external anal sphincter loses some of its ability to squeeze.

Aging can also bring other changes that may affect bowel function. Changes in the intestinal walls and blood supply slow down the time it takes for food and waste to move through your intestines. You might notice more constipation as stools become harder and drier.

Diseases that are common in older people, such as diabetes and Parkinson's disease, can contribute to fecal incontinence. In women, the effects of childbirth on the pelvic floor and anal muscles may become apparent only in their later years. Diet and lifestyle also have a great impact on how well your bowels work as you age. Older adults may drink fewer fluids because their sense of thirst is less acute. Older people who aren't physically active or who don't eat much fiber may have frequent constipation, which can lead to incontinence. Finally, some medications also contribute to fecal incontinence.

the vagina (rectocele) can be a cause of fecal incontinence. Hemorrhoids may prevent complete closure of the anal sphincter, leading to fecal incontinence.

Inability to hold stool (urge fecal incontinence)

When your external anal sphincter muscle isn't functioning properly, you may not be able to hold stool in — you feel urgency and must rush to the bathroom as soon as you sense stool in the rectum. You may not be able to squeeze the sphincter muscle hard enough or long enough to reach the toilet.

Childbirth is a common cause of anal sphincter damage. Giving birth vaginally can cause tears in both the internal and external anal sphincter muscles, as well as damage to the pudendal nerve, the major nerve to the external sphincter. Some women develop fecal incontinence within weeks of giving birth. For others, the problem doesn't show up until they're in their mid-40s or older, when muscles and supporting structures in the pelvis become weakened.

Other causes of anal sphincter damage include surgery for hemorrhoids, other rectal or anal operations, infections around the anal area, injury in the area and loss of strength in the muscles with increasing age. (See "Aging and fecal incontinence," on page 147.)

People with nerve damage in the pelvic floor may have problems with the rectum being able to accommodate stool. Stool passes through the sigmoid colon and rectum very quickly, and the barriers that normally hold stool in become overwhelmed. The result may be diarrhea or lack of time between sensing the presence of stool and an urgent need to use the bathroom. Such nerve damage may occur from diabetes, multiple sclerosis or spinal cord or brain injuries.

A sense of urgency and frequent bowel movements can also occur if your rectum can't stretch enough to store a normal amount of stool. Normally the rectum stretches to hold stool until you can get to a bathroom. But if your rectum can't stretch as much, you'll have less time between sensing the presence of stool and the urgent need to use the bathroom. Even if your sphincter muscles are working properly, you may experience fecal incontinence if your rectum has become stiff. Reduced rectal storage capacity can occur as a result of scarring from surgery, pelvic radiation or IBD.

A condition called rectal prolapse can make you feel an urgent need to go even when little stool is present. Rectal prolapse happens when the muscles supporting the rectum are weak, and the rectum prolapses — shifts downward into the anal canal or out of the body. If you have rectal prolapse, your external sphincter must work harder to hold stool in. Prolapse can cause sphincter damage, and most people with the condition experience fecal incontinence.

Impaired ability to sense stool (unsensed fecal incontinence)
Rectal sensation tells you that stool is in your rectum, and you need to get to a bathroom. If the nerves that are responsible for sensation in your rectum or anus are damaged, you may lose the ability to sense stool in your rectum. Or you may not be able to distinguish between gas, solid stool and liquid stool.

If rectal sensation is impaired, a person may not recognize the need to have a bowel movement. You may pass stool involuntarily, or excessive stool may accumulate in the rectum. This can cause impacted stool, hard fecal matter that's stuck in the rectum. Liquid stool eventually leaks out around the hard, impacted stool — this is known as overflow incontinence (see page 150).

Causes of impaired rectal sensation include nerve damage from diabetes, multiple sclerosis, stroke and spinal cord injury. Nerve injury can also occur from childbirth or from years of hard straining to defecate. Some medications, such as opiate painkillers and antidepressants, also can affect rectal sensation and lead to fecal incontinence. Rectal sensation may be blunted in older adults and physically and mentally challenged individuals.

Damage to your internal anal sphincter muscle also can lead to bits of stool leaking out without you being aware of it. A poor "seal" in the muscle allows stool to leak. If the sphincter sampling reflex is impaired, you may not be able to determine the contents of the rectum and decide what to do. The same things that can damage the external anal sphincter — childbirth, injury, surgery, muscle weakness with age — can also cause problems with the internal sphincter.

The ability to sense stool in the rectum also requires that a person is alert enough to notice the sensation and do something about it. A person with dementia may not notice the sensation, while a person with arthritis may have trouble getting to the bathroom. Fecal incontinence is often an aspect of late-stage Alzheimer's disease, in which both dementia and nerve damage play a role. Being physically disabled for any reason can make it difficult to reach a toilet in time.

Constipation and overflow incontinence

The most common cause of bowel incontinence, ironically, is constipation. Constipation is defined as passing stools less frequently than every three days, or excessive straining when trying to move the bowels. While many people believe that they should have at least one bowel movement a day, frequency varies from one person to another. If you pass at least three stools a week without straining, you're probably not constipated.

Like fecal incontinence, constipation is a sign of a problem, not a specific disease. Almost everyone becomes constipated at one time or another. Changes in your daily routine, such as travel, or changes in your diet can disrupt your bowel habits, leaving you constipated. Other possible causes of constipation include:

- Lack of physical activity
- Lack of dietary fiber
- Pregnancy and childbirth
- Diabetes and other hormone-related diseases
- Certain medications
- Surgery
- Irritable bowel syndrome
- Hemorrhoids
- Repeatedly ignoring the urge to defecate
- Diseases that affect the nerves, such as multiple sclerosis, stroke, dementia and Parkinson's disease
- Rectal prolapse and rectocele

Chronic constipation may lead to fecal impaction (impacted stool) — a large mass of dry, hard stool within the rectum. The mass may be too large for you to pass. The impacted, or stuck, stool causes your internal anal sphincter muscle to stretch and weaken. Watery stool from higher in the bowel may move around the mass and leak out. This type of incontinence is referred to as overflow incontinence. It can look like diarrhea, but anti-diarrheal medications will only make the problem worse.

Irritable bowel syndrome and incontinence

Irritable bowel syndrome (IBS) is characterized by abdominal pain or cramping and changes in bowel pattern, such as loose or more frequent bowel movements, diarrhea and constipation. About 20 percent of people with IBS report fecal incontinence.

It's not completely clear what causes IBS, but symptoms appear to result from a disturbance in the interaction between the intestines, the brain and the part of your nervous system that enables involuntary responses (autonomic nervous system). The result is a colon that's more sensitive and reactive to things such as stress and certain foods.

Up to one in five people in the United States has IBS. For most people, signs and symptoms are mild. Stress can aggravate symptoms. IBS can cause frequent diarrhea and constipation, both of which can lead to fecal incontinence. IBS can also lead to reduced storage capacity and sensation in the rectum.

For some people with IBS, the muscle contractions that move food through the digestive tract may be stronger and last longer than normal. Food is forced through your intestines more quickly, causing gas, bloating and diarrhea. This type of IBS, called diarrhea-predominant IBS, primarily affects men. Women are more likely to have the opposite problem — food passage slows, and stools become hard and dry, causing constipation. This is known as constipation-predominant IBS.

Some people have alternating bouts of constipation and diarrhea. You may also feel a sense of straining, urgency or a feeling that you can't empty your bowels completely.

A hopeful outlook

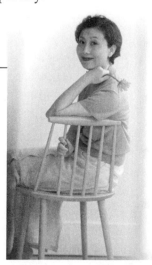

Many people aren't aware that effective treatments are available for fecal incontinence. You don't have to suffer in silence. Several different solutions address the various causes of incontinence. Treatment can improve your bowel control, and coping strategies can make living with incontinence a little easier.

Working up the courage to admit that you have incontinence is the first step in managing it. The following chapters provide information about getting help for fecal incontinence and about the different types of treatments.

Chapter 10

Getting help for fecal incontinence

M any people who live with fecal incontinence typically carry an added burden of shame and secrecy. They're embarrassed to tell a doctor about the problem. They may not realize that fecal incontinence is treatable, or they've had a bad experience with a doctor who didn't provide useful solutions or compassionate care.

They may try to cope on their own — buying adult diapers, memorizing every toilet facility in a given area, bringing a change of clothes every time they go out. These strategies work to a degree, but if you rely only on them, you may miss out on more effective treatments. Not getting help can result in needless suffering.

Don't shy away from talking to your doctor about fecal incontinence. Many treatments — some of which are very simple — are available that can improve, if not cure, incontinence. Nearly everyone can be helped in some way.

Taking that first step may well bring up some difficult feelings. It's common to feel embarrassed and anxious. Many people are angry or frustrated with the medical community for a lack of compassion and communication about the topic. These feelings are normal, and it's OK to express them.

Keep in mind that to your doctor, fecal incontinence isn't a personal problem or a reflection of your abilities, control or worth. It's a medical problem that can be investigated and treated. Ideally, your doctor will be your ally as you work together to find the best approach to your condition.

Choosing a doctor

To get help for fecal incontinence, your primary care doctor is a good place to start. Not all primary care doctors are familiar with evaluating and treating fecal incontinence, though. You may need to see someone who specializes in treating conditions that affect the colon, rectum and anus. Several types of health care professionals and clinics work with people who have fecal incontinence. These include:

Gastroenterologist. This type of doctor is trained to treat conditions of the digestive (gastrointestinal) tract, including fecal incontinence. If you have diarrhea or digestive symptoms in addition to incontinence, consider seeing a gastroenterologist.

Colorectal surgeon. Formerly known as a proctologist, this type of doctor provides surgical and nonsurgical treatment for diseases that affect the colon, rectum and anus.

Urogynecologist (female pelvic medicine and reconstructive surgery specialist). This type of doctor is a gynecologist who's had an additional three years of training in diseases and disorders affecting a woman's bladder and pelvis, including urinary and fecal incontinence.

Anorectal physiology lab. This facility specializes in evaluating people with fecal incontinence. The lab has trained clinicians and the necessary equipment for performing tests used to investigate possible causes of fecal incontinence.

What to expect

When you meet with a doctor to talk about fecal incontinence, it's important to feel comfortable. You have the right to be treated with dignity and respect. If the doctor seems to dismiss your problem, suggests that you use pads or tells you there's not much that can be done, find another physician.

Ask your doctor about his or her experience in treating fecal incontinence and about the range of treatments available. Not all doctors are aware that the problem is often correctable. Look for a practitioner who listens to your concerns, answers your questions and explains things clearly. He or she should show concern about how incontinence is affecting your quality of life.

Evaluating fecal incontinence

Your initial discussion with your doctor can help establish the degree and frequency of incontinence and its impact on your life. The doctor will likely ask many health-related questions and do a physical examination. This evaluation can help determine the cause of the incontinence and what tests may be needed to confirm the diagnosis. An accurate understanding of the cause or causes of fecal incontinence is essential for planning treatment.

Patient history

To help discover what might be causing your fecal incontinence, your doctor will likely ask many detailed questions about your symptoms, medical history and lifestyle. A careful medical history can provide many clues about the origins of incontinence. (See "Questions you may be asked during your exam," on page 156.) Some doctors use a standardized questionnaire or form to gather information and grade the severity of the incontinence.

The questions help determine whether you have true fecal incontinence and how severe it is. Expect questions about when the incontinence started, how often it occurs, whether the stool is liquid or solid, and whether you're aware of the need to go to the bathroom before the incontinence occurs. You may be asked to describe your normal bowel habits.

If you're a woman, you'll probably be asked about your history of childbirth, including the length of your labors, how much the babies weighed, whether you had a breech birth, whether the deliveries required forceps or episiotomies, whether you had any tears that needed repair, and how your bowels functioned after delivery.

Questions you may be asked during your exam

During the initial evaluation for fecal incontinence, your doctor will likely ask a lot of detailed questions about your bowel habits. Although you may find it embarrassing to reveal such personal information, it can help point toward what's causing the problem and what tests may be needed.

Be prepared to answer the following questions:
- When did the incontinence start?
- How often do you lose control of your bowels? What happens — do you lose a small or large amount of stool? Is it liquid or solid? Do you have any warning?
- Do you know when your rectum is full? Are you able to distinguish between gas and stool? Do you sometimes think you're passing gas and then are surprised to find that stool has come out?
- Does anything seem to bring on the incontinence, such as physical activity, illness, stress or specific foods? Does anything seem to make it better or worse?
- Has the problem gotten worse over time? Did it start after a particular event, such as surgery or childbirth?
- Do you experience incontinence at certain times of the day?

Your doctor may ask you if you also experience urinary incontinence, since urinary and fecal incontinence are sometimes related. He or she may want to know if you've had surgery, injuries or radiation treatment in your pelvic region or any back or spinal cord injuries. You'll also be asked about any other medical conditions you have, such as diabetes or irritable bowel syndrome.

Tell your doctor about any medications you take. Certain medications may cause or increase the frequency of bowel incontinence. Your doctor may also ask you about your diet and how much caffeine you consume.

It's important to talk about how you're coping with the incontinence and how it affects your daily life, relationships and self-esteem. Let your doctor know if you've made adjustments in your behavior or lifestyle, such as using pads, carrying a change of

Does it happen only at night or during the day? After meals? After a bowel movement?

- When you feel the need to have a bowel movement, how long can you wait?
- After you defecate, do you feel like there's stool left inside?
- What are your regular bowel habits? Were there changes in your bowel habits over the years?
- Do you often have diarrhea or constipation? Do you have to strain to pass stool? Is there any discomfort? Do you have cramps or see blood in your stool?
- Do you also experience urinary incontinence?
- Do you use pads or other devices to cope with incontinence? How is that working?
- Do you use anything to help with bowel movements, such as laxatives, enemas or suppositories?
- What medications are you taking?
- What is your typical diet?
- How does incontinence affect your life and how you feel about yourself?

clothes or not going out much to avoid the embarrassment of losing bowel control.

Your doctor may ask you to keep a diary of your symptoms and bowel habits. (See page 198 for an example of a bowel diary that you can copy and use.) Some items that might be recorded include bowel movements, incontinence episodes, the consistency of the stool, any feelings of straining, discomfort or incomplete emptying, and use of enemas or laxatives.

Physical exam

In addition to talking with you, your doctor will usually perform a physical examination. A careful physical exam can identify an injury or structural problem in the anal and rectal area, such as rectal prolapse, fecal impaction or rectocele. It can also help determine if fecal incontinence is caused by another disease, such as an ulcer or tumor, or from nerve damage caused by diseases such as diabetes or Parkinson's.

To check for signs of neurological disease or damage, your reflexes, walking gait and senses may be checked. Your doctor may also feel your abdomen. Swelling, tenderness or pain in your abdomen may indicate gas, fluid or a blockage of some kind in your colon.

A rectal examination is necessary to evaluate fecal incontinence. Some people consider this exam uncomfortable and undignified. But the information it provides is key to diagnosing the problem.

The rectal exam starts with a visual inspection of your anus and the area between your anus and genitals, called the perineum. Your doctor looks for fecal matter, hemorrhoids, reddening, scarring and signs of infection. Your buttocks are gently spread apart, and the shape of your anus is checked — open or closed, round or asymmetrical, intact or cracked.

Sensation in the area between your anus and genitals also is checked. Using a pin, probe or cotton swab, your doctor gently touches various points around your anus to see if it puckers up — a "winking" reflex that occurs as the anal sphincter contracts. This test helps check for nerve damage.

The doctor may also perform a digital rectal exam (DRE). He or she inserts a gloved, lubricated finger into your rectum to evaluate the strength of your sphincter muscles and to feel for hemorrhoids, growths, tears, protrusions or scars. This exam also can usually identify fecal impaction, a large mass of dry, hard stool within your rectum. Impaction can lead to overflow incontinence, in which watery stool leaks out around the mass of stool. (See page 46 for an illustration of a DRE.)

During the DRE, you'll be asked to squeeze your muscles around the doctor's finger and bear down as if you were trying to have a bowel movement. This can help the doctor feel whether the rectal sphincter muscles and the puborectalis muscle in your pelvic floor are working — is there a resting muscle tone, can you generate an extra squeeze, can you relax your muscles, do the muscles keep the colon and rectum at the proper angle?

The DRE exam can also help identify rectal prolapse, a condition in which the rectum drops down into the anus. If your doctor suspects rectal prolapse, he or she may ask you to sit upright on a toilet and strain and lean forward while he or she inspects your anal area.

If you feel any pain during the rectal exam, tell your doctor. The exam may be uncomfortable but shouldn't be painful.

Tests to evaluate fecal incontinence

Using the findings of the medical history and physical exam, your doctor may determine a working diagnosis and recommend conservative initial treatment, such as changes in diet, medications or fluid intake, simple pelvic floor exercises, or anti-diarrheal medications. (See Chapter 11 for more information about treatment for fecal incontinence.)

Often, however, more information is needed to pinpoint the cause of fecal incontinence and help plan treatment. In this case, you may be scheduled for tests.

A number of tests are available to more completely investigate the causes of incontinence. Imaging tests provide a visual picture of the lower colon, rectum and anus. Functional tests assess how well these parts of the body are working. Which tests are done depends on your symptoms and the information your doctor gains from your medical history and physical exam.

Manometry

Manometry (muh-NOM-uh-tre), also called anal manometry or anorectal manometry, is the most commonly used test for evaluating fecal incontinence. Manometry is also used in biofeedback treatment. (See "Biofeedback," on page 57.)

This test measures the pressure inside your rectum and anal sphincters. It checks the strength of your anal sphincter muscles and their ability to relax and tighten at the proper times. It also evaluates the sensitivity and function of your rectum.

The test may be done in your doctor's office or at a clinic or hospital. It takes about 30 minutes to an hour. As you're lying on your side, your doctor inserts a narrow, flexible tube (about the circumference of a rectal thermometer) into your anus and rectum. The tube has a small, deflated balloon at the end. Once the tube is in place, the balloon may be expanded.

The balloon senses the pressure inside your rectum, your internal anal sphincter and your external anal sphincter and transmits the data to a computer. The results are displayed on a graph that looks something like that of a polygraph. Pressure measurements are recorded as you rest, squeeze and bear down as if trying to pass stool. An abnormally low sphincter pressure indicates a problem with the muscle. Decreased pressure when you're resting or relaxed suggests a problem with the internal anal sphincter, and decreased pressure when you're squeezing suggests that the external anal sphincter isn't working properly.

Manometry is also used to check sensation in your rectum. The ability to sense stool in your rectum is critical for being able to know when you need to go to the bathroom. The test also evaluates how well your rectum expands and contracts when stool enters it (rectal compliance).

Your doctor may ask you to close your eyes as the balloon is inflated. As the balloon fills with air or fluid, the doctor will ask if you can feel it. He or she will ask when you feel the first sensation in your rectum, when you feel an urge to defecate and when the sensation starts to feel urgent. The computer records the changes in pressure in your rectum as the balloon is expanded to different levels. This reflects the rectum's ability to stretch.

Occasionally other tests may be done during manometry to assess how well your bowels are working. Two simple tests are balloon expulsion and saline infusion.

Balloon expulsion. This test evaluates your basic ability to defecate — the ability of your puborectalis muscle to relax and the coordination of your abdominal, pelvic floor and anal sphincter muscles. Most people with fecal incontinence are able to have normal bowel movements, but people whose fecal incontinence or seepage is caused by chronic constipation and impacted stool may have trouble passing stool normally. The test simply involves expelling the balloon that's been placed in your rectum.

If you have diarrhea or constipation

If you have diarrhea along with fecal incontinence, your doctor may ask you for a stool sample. It will be tested in the laboratory for bacteria or other organisms that may be causing infection. Your doctor may also want to examine your rectum and colon using a flexible viewing tube, or scope, to make sure the diarrhea isn't caused by inflammation in the colon or a mass in the rectum. (See "Looking inside the colon and rectum," on page 162.)

If you're experiencing ongoing constipation, your doctor may perform colon transit studies. These tests check whether digestive contents are moving through your colon too slowly. To prepare, stop taking all laxatives three days before the test. The procedure involves swallowing a slightly radioactive tracer substance that follows the journey from mouth to anus. The markers can be seen in X-rays to show how long it takes them to travel through the digestive tract.

Saline infusion. This test is meant to "stress" the anal sphincters by simulating conditions similar to diarrhea. A saltwater solution or other substance is put into your rectum. The test shows whether your sphincters are able to maintain continence with the fluid in your rectum. People who don't have fecal incontinence usually retain most of the liquid, but people with fecal incontinence, particularly those whose rectal capacity is limited or impaired, leak sooner.

Ultrasound

This technique uses sound waves to create images of the internal and external anal sphincters. Anal ultrasound is used to evaluate the structure of the anal sphincters and can identify defects, scarring, thinning or other abnormalities in these muscles. It's a simple, reliable and inexpensive procedure.

Commonly known as ultrasound, this imaging test may be referred to by various names — endoanal ultrasonography, endorectal ultrasonography, anorectal ultrasonography and endosonography. In an endoscopic ultrasound test, a probe that

Looking inside the colon and rectum

Your doctor may want to use a viewing tube to take a closer look at your anus, rectum and colon. This enables him or her to see signs of disease or other problems that could cause fecal incontinence, such as inflammation, a tumor, scar tissue or rectal prolapse. The doctor will look for changes in the lining of your colon and rectum that might reflect damage to underlying nerves and muscles. Visual examination is also useful for evaluating diarrhea, constipation or other changes in bowel habits.

Two procedures are used to view the colon and rectum — proctosigmoidoscopy and colonoscopy. Together the tests are referred to as lower gastrointestinal endoscopy. Colonoscopy isn't usually necessary for evaluating fecal incontinence, but your doctor may suggest it if your symptoms point to the possibility of colorectal cancer or another disease of the colon.

Both tests use a long, slender tube with a tiny video camera and light on the end. The tube is attached to a video monitor. The camera provides a clear, detailed view of the lining of the colon and rectum. The doctor can see bleeding, inflammation, abnormal growths or ulcers.

For proctosigmoidoscopy, your doctor uses a tube called a sigmoidoscope to examine your rectum and sigmoid colon, and perhaps part of your descending colon. (See image on the next page.) Colonoscopy is performed using a colonoscope, a tube that's long enough to inspect the full length of the large intestine and part of the small intestine.

Your colon and rectum must be completely empty during these procedures. The night before, you'll be asked to drink only clear liquids, and you won't be able to eat or drink anything after midnight. You'll cleanse your bowels by taking a laxative or having an enema.

The test is done on an outpatient basis at a hospital or in your doctor's office. A proctosigmoidoscopy takes 10 to 20 minutes. A colonoscopy takes 30 minutes to an hour. For a colonoscopy, you'll be given medication to make you relaxed and drowsy.

For both exams, you'll lie on your left side on an examining table. The doctor will gently insert the well-lubricated scope into your rectum and slowly guide it into your colon. You may feel as if you need to move your bowels as the scope is advanced. The scope can be used to blow air into the colon and rectum to inflate them, which allows for a better view of the lining. You may feel some cramping or fullness as this happens.

If your doctor discovers anything unusual in your colon, such as a small growth on the lining of the colon (polyp) or inflamed tissue, he or she may remove a piece of it using instruments inserted into the scope. The tissue sample (biopsy) can be tested for cell abnormalities.

After the test, you can get back to your usual diet and activities right away. You may pass gas or feel some mild bloating or cramping. These symptoms usually disappear within a day.

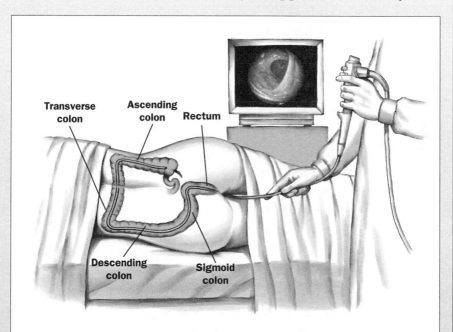

During colonoscopy a thin, flexible tube is inserted into your rectum and threaded through your colon (large intestine). Images from inside the lower gastrointestinal tract appear on a video monitor.

emits sound waves is placed on the tip of a flexible, lighted viewing tube called an endoscope.

The ultrasound probe, which is attached to a computer and video screen, is inserted through your anus and into your rectum. The waves bounce off the walls of your rectum and anus, producing video images of these internal structures. The doctor can see how your sphincter muscles move and whether any part of them is torn, missing or too thin.

Anal ultrasound is most useful for identifying sphincter injuries or defects and ruling out other muscle or nerve damage as the cause of incontinence. If your medical history suggests that you may have a tear or other problem in the anal sphincters, your doctor will likely recommend this test.

Anal electromyography

If the nerves that control your anal sphincter muscles are damaged, they may not work properly, leading to fecal incontinence. Fecal incontinence is often the result of both muscle and nerve damage. For example, childbirth can injure the pudendal nerve — the major nerve supplying the external anal sphincter — as well as the sphincter muscles.

Anal electromyography (EMG) can assess whether nerve damage is causing or contributing to fecal incontinence. The test is useful for people who have an underlying disease, such as diabetes, that may cause nerve damage, or if your doctor believes that you may have pelvic floor nerve damage from childbirth, surgery or an injury. Assessing the level of nerve damage can help determine whether surgery is likely to be helpful.

Anal EMG records electrical activity within your anal sphincter muscles. For this test, a small sponge containing an electrode is inserted into your anus. It's similar to having a digital rectal exam, with the addition of the sponge electrode attached to your doctor's gloved finger. As you squeeze and relax your sphincter muscles, the electrode will record their electrical signals.

Less commonly, the test may be done with tiny needle electrodes inserted into muscles around your anus. But the needle procedure isn't performed often, since it's quite painful.

Pudendal nerve stimulation

This test — called pudendal nerve terminal motor latency, or PNTML — is similar to anal EMG. It records electrical activity in the pudendal nerve to test for damage to the nerve. An injured pudendal nerve can result in weakness in the anal sphincter muscles. PNTML may be used with anal ultrasound or manometry to determine whether incontinence is caused by nerve damage, muscle damage or both.

In this test, as in anal EMG, a small electrode is inserted into your anal canal. The electrode delivers a mild electrical current to the pudendal nerve. The amount of time it takes for the sphincter muscle to contract in response to the current is measured. You may feel a slight vibration during the test.

Magnetic resonance imaging

Magnetic resonance imaging (MRI) uses a magnet and radio waves to create detailed, layered (cross-sectional) images of body tissues — in this case, the anal sphincter muscles and surrounding area. MRI is more expensive than are other tests and may not offer advantages over tests such as anal ultrasound. A newer form of MRI called dynamic MRI has shown promise in evaluating problems with the pelvic floor, rectum and anus.

For a traditional MRI, you lie very still on a table that's rolled into the opening of a large, tunnel-shaped magnet. Some MRI machines have an open scanner that doesn't require you to be in an enclosed space.

Before the test, a contrast dye will be given to you in a vein (intravenously). The dye shows the response of body tissues to being in a magnetic field and allows the MRI machine to create images of the inside of the body. To get a clearer picture of your anal sphincters, a slim coil or tube may be inserted in your rectum.

Dynamic MRI creates a real-time image of your pelvic floor as you move your bowels, allowing the doctor to see any abnormalities that occur as you defecate. For this test, your rectum is filled with ultrasound gel, and while you're lying in the MRI machine you pass the gel out as if it were stool. The machine creates a series of images of the defecation process.

Preliminary research indicates that dynamic MRI is useful for identifying anal sphincter problems, pelvic floor problems, such as rectal prolapse, and rectocele.

Defecography

This test shows how much and how well your rectum can hold stool and how well your rectum works during defecation. Like dynamic MRI, it provides a visual picture of the dynamics of defecation. Defecography may be useful for evaluating suspected rectal prolapse or other problems or if you're having trouble completely emptying your rectum.

In this procedure, your doctor inserts a small amount of barium paste into your rectum. Barium coats the walls of your rectum and makes it visible on X-rays. The paste has a similar consistency to that of stool. You'll sit on a specially designed seat similar to a toilet. Motion in your pelvic floor can be recorded on video or X-rays as you rest, cough, squeeze and strain to pass the barium out of your rectum.

How the tests are used

The test results, along with your symptoms and history, help your doctor develop a working diagnosis and choose appropriate treatment. The test results also can provide your doctor with much more information about the appearance and function of your bowels.

Once the testing has been done and your doctor has a working diagnosis, you and your doctor can begin discussing a treatment plan. Fortunately, effective treatments are available for fecal incontinence that can improve your quality of life.

Chapter 11

Treating fecal incontinence

S eeking help for fecal incontinence is the first step in managing it. Acknowledging the problem and working with a sympathetic, supportive doctor can ease some of the feelings of isolation, embarrassment and depression that many people with fecal incontinence experience.

Fortunately, effective treatments are available for fecal incontinence. Treatment usually can help restore bowel control or at least substantially reduce the severity of symptoms. An important goal of treatment is to improve your quality of life. Various coping strategies can make living with fecal incontinence easier.

Treatment depends on the cause of your incontinence and how severe it is. Treatment normally starts with nonsurgical options. These may include changing your diet, regulating your bowel habits, using biofeedback or taking a medication. For many people, the simplest treatments provide substantial relief. If conservative approaches don't work, surgery may be recommended.

Because incontinence often results from more than one cause, more than one form of treatment may be needed for successful bowel control. Your doctor can also address any medical conditions that may be contributing to incontinence, such as impacted stool, dementia, neurological problems, inflammatory bowel disease and lactose intolerance.

Behavioral treatments

Treating fecal incontinence often begins with steps to modify your behavior and habits. These behavioral approaches may be all that's necessary to bring incontinence under control, or they may be combined with other treatments. Almost everyone can gain some benefit from behavioral treatments. Studies have concluded that conservative treatment not only helps with fecal incontinence but also improves quality of life, psychological well-being and anal sphincter function. You can also feel more in control by developing better coping strategies for dealing with incontinence episodes that do occur.

Diet

Diet has a major effect on bowel function. What you eat and drink affects the consistency of your stool and how quickly it passes through the digestive system. Changes to your diet can improve your bowel movements and make them more predictable.

Your doctor will help you find a diet that helps you gain good stool consistency. You'll also want to avoid foods that irritate your system. Following are some dietary factors that may affect your bowel control.

Fiber. Foods that are high in fiber can help improve the consistency of stool, making it softer, bulkier and more formed. A soft, bulky stool is easier to pass than a hard, small stool. Formed stool is also less likely to leak out than more watery stool. A fiber-rich diet promotes more frequent and regular bowel movements and can help control both constipation and diarrhea.

Fiber, also known as roughage or bulk, includes all parts of plant foods that your body can't digest or absorb. It's found mainly in fruits, vegetables, whole grains and legumes.

Insoluble fiber doesn't dissolve in water. It moves through your digestive system quickly, making the stool bulkier. It's found in bananas, brown rice, tapioca, whole-grain bread, potatoes, applesauce, cheese, yogurt, pasta and oatmeal. Soluble fiber dissolves in water to form a soft, gel-like material in the intestines. This type of fiber is found in oat bran, beans, barley, nuts, seeds, lentils, peas, apples, citrus fruits and carrots.

So how much fiber should you eat? Experts recommend 20 to 30 grams a day, but adding too much fiber to your diet all at once can cause bloating, gas or diarrhea. Too much insoluble fiber can also contribute to diarrhea. If eating more fiber seems to make your diarrhea worse, cut back to two servings each of fruits and vegetables a day. Removing the skins and seeds from your food also can help.

When you increase your fiber intake, it's important to drink plenty of water. Fiber works best when it absorbs water. Without enough fluids, the stool becomes hard and can lead to constipation.

Good sources of fiber include raw or cooked fruits and vegetables, whole-grain breads and cereals, brown rice, and dried beans and peas. Other sources of dietary fiber are listed in "High fiber foods" on pages 170-171.

You can also boost your fiber intake with supplements such as Metamucil, Citrucel and FiberCon, which help move water into the bowel and propel stool toward the rectum. Supplements can increase stool volume and reduce watery stools. They may be helpful for some people, but can worsen diarrhea or incontinence in others. Supplements also don't provide the vitamins and other nutrients found in high-fiber foods. Talk to your doctor about whether a supplement is appropriate for you.

Increasing fiber intake isn't helpful for everyone. Older adults who are inactive may have more problems with incontinence if they eat a high-fiber diet. For people with constipation that's due to a slowed-down digestive system, too much fiber can cause bloating and abdominal pain.

Drinks and foods with caffeine. Coffee and other caffeine-containing drinks and foods can act as laxatives, causing diarrhea or an urgent need to use the toilet. Reducing your caffeine consumption, especially after meals, can help lessen the sense of urgency and diarrhea. A list of foods that may worsen fecal incontinence appears on pages 190-191 of the Appendix.

Meal size and times. In some people, large meals can cause bowel contractions that lead to diarrhea. You can avoid this by eating several small meals throughout the day rather than three large ones. In general, eating regularly timed, well-balanced meals will help with bowel regularity.

High-fiber foods

Here's a look at the fiber content of some common foods. Read nutrition labels to find out how much fiber is in your favorite foods.

Fruits	Serving size	Total fiber (grams)
Pear	1 medium	5.1
Raspberries	1/2 cup	4.0
Figs, dried	2 medium	3.7
Blueberries	1 cup	3.5
Apple, with skin	1 medium	3.3
Peaches, dried	3 halves	3.3
Orange	1 medium	3.1
Strawberries	1 cup	3.0
Apricots, dried	10 halves	2.6
Raisins	1 1/2-ounce box	1.6

Grains, cereals and pastas	Serving size	Total fiber (grams)
Spaghetti, whole-wheat	1 cup	6.3
Bran flakes	3/4 cup	5.3
Oatmeal	1 cup	4.0
Bread, rye	1 slice	1.9
Bread, whole-wheat	1 slice	1.9
Bread, mixed-grain	1 slice	1.7
Bread, cracked-wheat	1 slice	1.4

Fluids. To prevent dehydration and keep your stools soft and formed, drink plenty of water and other liquids. Fluids help foods move through the digestive system and keep you from getting constipated.

Try to drink eight 8-ounce glasses of water a day (unless you have a medical condition requiring you to restrict your fluid intake). Avoid caffeine-containing beverages, alcohol, milk and carbonated drinks if you find that they contribute to diarrhea.

If you're prone to diarrhea or a feeling of urgency to use the toilet, you can slow down your digestive system by drinking at a dif-

Legumes, nuts and seeds	Serving size	Total fiber (grams)
Lentils	1 cup	15.6
Black beans	1 cup	15.0
Baked beans, canned	1 cup	13.9
Lima beans	1 cup	13.2
Almonds	24 nuts	3.3
Pistachio nuts	47 nuts	2.9
Peanuts	28 nuts	2.3
Cashews	18 nuts	0.9

Vegetables	Serving size	Total fiber (grams)
Peas	1 cup	8.8
Artichoke, cooked	1 medium	6.5
Brussels sprouts	1 cup	6.4
Turnip greens, boiled	1 cup	5.0
Potato, baked with skin	1 medium	4.4
Corn	1 cup	4.2
Broccoli, raw	1 medium stalk	4.0
Popcorn, air-popped	3 cups	3.6
Tomato paste	1/4 cup	3.0
Spinach, cooked	1 cup	2.0
Carrot	1 medium	1.8

Source: Department of Agriculture, National Nutrient Database for Standard Reference, 2004

ferent time from when you eat. For example, have a glass of water or other beverage before or after a meal but not with meals.

Medications that can cause fecal incontinence

Some medications that you may take for other conditions can contribute to fecal incontinence. Your doctor may suggest a change in your medications if they're causing diarrhea, constipation or incontinence. Be sure to tell your doctor about any medications and vitamin and mineral supplements you're taking. Their possible effects on your continence will be evaluated. (A list of medications that

Controlling gas

Even as your bowel control improves, you'll still pass gas. That's normal. Everyone has gas in the digestive tract. As with incontinence, changes in diet can help control excessive gas.

Gas in the digestive tract comes from two main sources — swallowed air and the normal breakdown of undigested food in the large intestine. Most foods that contain carbohydrates can cause gas. Gas-producing foods include:

- Beans
- Some vegetables, such as asparagus, broccoli, cabbage, brussels sprouts, cauliflower, cucumbers, green peppers, onions and radishes
- Some fruits, such as apples, peaches and pears
- Whole grains and bran
- Carbonated drinks
- Milk and milk products
- Packaged foods made with lactose, such as bread, cereal and salad dressing
- Foods with sorbitol, such as sugar-free candies and gums

can contribute to fecal incontinence or make it worse appears on pages 194-195 of the Appendix.)

Bowel regulation and control

Establishing regular bowel habits is a simple approach that can make a big difference in managing incontinence. Bowel retraining can help some people relearn how to control their bowels. It can also help restore muscle strength if your fecal incontinence stems from a lack of anal sphincter control or decreased awareness of the urge to defecate.

A program of bowel retraining involves several steps and strategies aimed at producing regular bowel movements. In some cases, bowel retraining means going to the toilet at set times of the day. In other cases, the training involves exercise therapy.

Some people achieve bowel control by making a conscious effort to have bowel movements at specific times during the day, such

Foods that are more likely to form odorous gas include alcohol, asparagus, beans, cabbage, chicken, coffee, cucumbers, dairy products, eggs, fish, garlic, nuts, onions, prunes and radishes.

If gas is a problem, keep a food diary for a week or so to identify what foods may cause gas or affect its odor. Many of the foods that cause gas, such as fruits, vegetables and whole grains, are important parts of a healthy diet, so the solution isn't to cut them out altogether. Experiment to find out how much of the offending foods you can handle.

In addition, several over-the-counter medications can help reduce symptoms. These include antacids with simethicone (Gas-X, Mylanta Gas, Phazyme), activated charcoal tablets (CharcoCaps, Charcoal Plux) and Beano. If you have problems with milk and other dairy products, the enzyme lactase can help you digest lactose, the sugar in milk. Lactase is available in liquid and tablet form, or you can buy lactose-reduced milk and other products.

as after every meal. This helps you gain greater control by establishing some predictability about when you use the toilet. It can be especially helpful for people whose fecal incontinence is caused by constipation.

Before you start any bowel-retraining program, your doctor will want to make sure you don't have fecal impaction. The impacted stool must be removed before bowel training can work. (See "Treating stool impaction" on page 175.)

To help develop a regular pattern of bowel movements, consider these tips:

- Establish a set time for daily bowel movements. Choose times that are convenient for you, keeping in mind your daily schedule and your past patterns of elimination. The best time for a bowel movement is 20 to 30 minutes after a meal because eating stimulates bowel activity and your rectum is likely to be full, even if you don't feel a need to go. The goal is to establish a routine and predictable time for elimination — the same time each day.

• If you have constipation or irritable bowel syndrome, it may take some time before you're able to go "on demand." To establish a routine, try sitting on the toilet for a few minutes, even if you don't feel like you need to go or if you don't actually have a bowel movement. With practice your bowels may be stimulated to work more effectively. However, sitting too long may contribute to the development of hemorrhoids. If you're unsuccessful after a few minutes, it's usually better to get up and walk around a bit, then try again.

• Some people find it helpful to drink a hot drink or warm prune juice to stimulate a bowel movement.

• Your doctor may recommend that you try stimulating a bowel movement by inserting a lubricated finger into your anus. Move your finger in a circular motion until the sphincter muscle relaxes. It might take a few minutes.

• Some people may need to use suppositories, enemas, laxatives or a combination of these to stimulate a bowel movement. These measures should be used only under your doctor's advice. It's best to use the least stimulation that's effective.

• Try to relax when you're on the toilet and assume a posture that's conducive to defecating. Avoid straining.

Persistence and consistency are the keys to success with this approach. It may take a while to form a regular pattern. Try not to get frustrated and give up if it doesn't happen right away. Most people can achieve regular bowel movements within a few weeks of starting a bowel program.

The training should be tailored to your individual condition. For example, if you have a rectal prolapse or rectocele, the focus may be on reducing the number of attempts to have a bowel movement and stopping excessive straining. In this case, you might be advised to attempt to have a bowel movement no more than three times a day.

Pelvic floor exercises. No matter what the cause of your fecal incontinence, your doctor may recommend exercises to strengthen your pelvic floor and sphincter and rectal muscles (Kegel exercises). These exercises can be combined with other treatments and are

---

Treating stool impaction

If you have a mass of hard stool in your rectum (impacted stool), the first line of treatment is to remove it. If taking laxatives or using enemas doesn't help you pass the mass, your doctor may have to assist in removing it. To do so, the doctor inserts one or two fingers into your rectum and breaks the impacted stool into fragments that you can then expel.

After the impacted stool is expelled, your doctor may suggest a number of steps to prevent constipation, such as increasing your intake of fiber and fluids and becoming more physically active. Other possible remedies include mild laxatives, stool softeners, enemas and suppositories.

---

used as part of biofeedback treatment. Pelvic floor muscle training is described in detail beginning on page 191 of the Appendix.

Biofeedback

Biofeedback is a way of giving you visual, audio or verbal feedback about a body function, such as muscle activity, that you normally don't perceive. As a treatment for fecal incontinence, biofeedback is used to help strengthen and coordinate the muscles involved in holding in stool. It can also improve your ability to sense the presence of stool in your rectum.

Many people with fecal incontinence gain at least some benefit from biofeedback. The technique may be useful if your incontinence is due to weak sphincter muscles, impaired rectal sensation, chronic constipation or nerve damage from diabetes, childbirth or surgery. But people with severe fecal incontinence or underlying neurological diseases may be less likely to benefit. In addition, biofeedback may not be a useful treatment for people with no or very limited rectal sensation.

Because biofeedback is safe and effective, it's often recommended before considering surgical treatment. Whether biofeedback will work for you depends on the cause of your incontinence and how severe the muscle or nerve damage is. Success also depends on your own motivation and the biofeedback therapist's expertise.

Physical activity and bowel health

One way to keep your bowels moving is to keep moving your body. Regular physical exercise stimulates intestinal muscle activity, helping to move food waste through your intestines. Lack of physical activity is a common cause of constipation in older adults and people whose mobility is limited because of stroke, spinal injury or another medical condition.

Staying physically active can help promote regular bowel movements and help prevent constipation. But if you're prone to diarrhea or have trouble holding in stool, brisk physical activity — particularly after meals or soon after waking up in the morning — may lead to incontinence.

Use a bowel symptom diary (see pages 198-199) to chart whether and when exercise triggers incontinence episodes for you. You may need to exercise at a different time of day or choose more moderate activities.

Techniques. One biofeedback technique involves inserting a pressure-sensitive probe into your anal canal. The probe registers the strength and activity of your anal sphincter muscle as it contracts around the probe. The practitioner will teach you how to squeeze your anal muscles around the probe. You can practice sphincter contractions and learn to strengthen your own muscles by viewing the scale's readout as a visual aid or by hearing audio responses to your muscle contractions. The feedback about how your muscles are working helps ensure that you're doing the exercises correctly and shows whether your muscles are getting stronger.

Another biofeedback technique uses manometry equipment to vary the pressure in your rectum (for more information on manometry, see page 159). In this procedure, a probe with a deflated balloon is inserted into your rectum. The practitioner will then inflate the balloon to various levels, training you to detect smaller amounts of stool in your rectum through the use of feedback. Another technique uses three balloons and teaches you to respond to sensation in your rectum by immediately and forcefully squeezing your anal sphincter muscle.

Results. A typical biofeedback program requires four to six sessions. Sometimes, one session is all you need. Most people see an improvement in symptoms after three sessions.

For the best results, it's important that you feel comfortable with your biofeedback therapist. You may have the treatment at a biofeedback clinic, at your doctor's office or at the office of a therapist trained in biofeedback. He or she will likely begin by asking a number of questions about your bowel habits and history. The therapist can also provide support, advice and education about your bowel habits.

In addition to training you to use your sphincter muscles, the therapist may also teach you techniques for proper defecation, as well as relaxation techniques, because many people with fecal incontinence become anxious when they feel the urge to go.

Coping strategies

Sometimes, fecal incontinence takes time to improve or is due to a problem that can't be completely corrected. You may not be able to avoid having an incontinent episode at times. Having a plan for these times helps lessen feelings of fear, embarrassment, anger, isolation, humiliation and loneliness.

Fear of having an accident may keep you from wanting to go out in public, work or attend social events. To overcome this fear, try these practical tips:

- Use the toilet before heading out.
- If you think an episode is likely while you're out, wear pads or disposable undergarments.
- Carry cleanup supplies and a change of clothing.
- Locate public restrooms before you need them and make sure you can get to them easily.
- Be flexible about plans. If you don't feel comfortable leaving the house on a particular day, change the plan to another day.

Self-care products. Products such as absorbent pads and disposable underwear can help you better manage incontinence, though it can be difficult to accept that you need them. You can purchase incontinence products at drugstores, supermarkets, medical supply stores or online.

Caring for someone with fecal incontinence

If you care for someone with fecal incontinence, try to be supportive and not critical. Consider these tips:

- Make regular trips to the bathroom with your loved one, to help him or her avoid an accident.
- Make sure clothing is easy to open or remove.
- Place a commode near the bed.
- Use washable cushions or slipcovers.
- Use absorbent undergarments and washable bed pads.
- Clean the skin around the person's anal area immediately after an incontinent episode. Follow the suggestions on this page for keeping the anal area clean and dry.

If you use pads or adult diapers, be sure they have an absorbent wicking layer on top. Products with this layer protect your skin by pulling stool and moisture away from skin and into the pad.

Relieving anal discomfort. The skin around your anus is delicate and sensitive. Diarrhea, constipation or contact between stool and skin can cause pain or itching. Consider the following practices to relieve anal discomfort and eliminate possible odor associated with fecal incontinence:

- Wash with water. Gently wash the area around your anus with plain water after each bowel movement, either by using wet toilet paper, showering or soaking in a bath. Soap can dry skin, worsening irritation. Avoid rubbing with dry toilet paper. Pre-moistened, alcohol-free towelettes are a good choice for cleaning the area.
- Dry thoroughly. Allow the area to air-dry after washing. If you don't have time, gently pat the area dry with clean toilet paper or a clean washcloth. Using a hair dryer may also help, but be sure it's set on the cool setting.
- Apply a cream or powder. Use a moisture-barrier cream to keep irritated skin from direct contact with stool. Ask your doctor to recommend a product. Be sure the area is clean before applying the cream. You can also try nonmedicated talcum powder or cornstarch to relieve anal discomfort.

- Wear cotton underwear and loose clothing. Tight clothing can restrict airflow and worsen anal problems. Change soiled underwear as soon as possible.
- If it helps you feel more comfortable, consider using a deodorant such as Periwash or Derifil.

Medications

Medications may be part of your treatment plan for fecal incontinence if you have loose, watery stools or diarrhea, or if chronic constipation is causing your fecal incontinence. Your doctor will try to identify and treat the underlying disorder that's causing diarrhea or constipation. If a disorder can't be found or corrected, you may be given a medication to relieve your signs and symptoms and restore bowel control.

Drugs to prevent diarrhea

As a first step in treating diarrhea or loose stools, your doctor may recommend that you include more high-fiber foods in your diet or that you take an over-the-counter anti-diarrheal agent such as activated attapulgite (Kaopectate, Diarrest, Diatrol). Stool softeners such as Metamucil, MiraLax and Citrucel also can help because they make stools bulkier and less fluid.

The anti-diarrheal drug most commonly used in treating fecal incontinence is loperamide (Imodium), which is also available without a prescription. Loperamide slows down bowel activity, reducing stool frequency and making stools more formed. The drug has the added benefit of increasing rectal and anal sensitivity, which also improves bowel control. Taking loperamide before going out for a meal or social occasion can help you avoid an incontinent episode in public.

Your doctor can help you determine the proper dose of loperamide. Side effects are generally mild but may include constipation, abdominal cramping, dry mouth and nausea.

Other anti-diarrheal medications that are sometimes used to treat fecal incontinence include diphenoxylate (Lofene, Logen,

Lomocot, Lomotil, Lonox, Vi-Atro), difenoxin (Motofen) and alos-etron (Lotronex).

Drugs for constipation

If chronic constipation is causing your incontinence, your doctor may recommend the temporary use of mild laxatives, such as milk of magnesia, to help restore normal bowel movements. To prevent stool impaction, your doctor may recommend a stool-softening supplement such as Metamucil, MiraLax or Citrucel.

The prescription medication tegaserod (Zelnorm) may be used as a short-term treatment for women with irritable bowel syndrome who have constipation as their main bowel problem, or for women under age 65 who have chronic constipation.

Other medications

There currently are no medications specifically approved for the treatment of fecal incontinence. Drugs used to treat inflammatory bowel disease are sometimes used to control fecal incontinence. Other drugs, including the nasal decongestant phenylephrine gel and the antidepressant drug amitriptyline, are being studied for their effects on fecal incontinence. If you have a question about medications, talk with your doctor.

Surgery

Most people with fecal incontinence don't need surgery. But if other treatments are unsuccessful and incontinence remains severe and disabling, surgical options may be considered. Surgery may be helpful for people whose incontinence is caused by damage to the pelvic floor, anal canal or anal sphincter, perhaps from a tear during childbirth, a fracture or a past operation.

Various surgical procedures can be done, ranging from repairs of damaged areas to complex surgeries to replace the anal sphincter with an artificial sphincter or with muscle from another part of the body. Surgery to treat fecal incontinence isn't free of complications. But it's often effective for certain causes of fecal incontinence.

Treating double incontinence

Many people experience both urinary and fecal incontinence, or double incontinence. The two conditions can stem from many of the same causes, including muscle and nerve damage from childbirth, years of straining to have bowel movements, muscular weakness with aging, and diseases that cause nerve damage.

If you have combined urinary and fecal incontinence, you may need to see more than one doctor or find someone who has experience in both areas. You might see a gynecologist, urogynecologist, urologist, colon and rectal surgeon, or gastroenterologist.

Treatment for double incontinence typically begins with behavior approaches, including pelvic floor muscle exercises, bladder and bowel training, and biofeedback. Surgery may be recommended to repair both an anal sphincter defect and pelvic floor problems. Early studies of a new treatment, sacral nerve stimulation (see pages 184-185), show some promise for people who have fecal incontinence along with urinary urge incontinence.

Sphincteroplasty

Sphincteroplasty is surgery to repair a damaged or weakened anal sphincter. It's the most common surgical procedure used to treat fecal incontinence. The operation is effective for people who have a single site of anal sphincter injury, such as a tear that occurred during vaginal delivery. A tear or interruption in the ring of muscle that makes up the external anal sphincter keeps it from closing tightly enough to hold stool in.

During a sphincteroplasty, the surgeon identifies the injured area of muscle and frees its edges from the surrounding tissue. The muscle edges are then brought back and sewn together in an overlapping fashion to create a complete ring of muscle, restoring the anus to its proper shape. This strengthens the muscle and tightens the sphincter.

A colon and rectal surgeon, urogynecologist, or gynecologic surgeon usually performs this surgery. You'll likely be in the hospital for several days, and it may be a month or more before you return to your usual activities. You'll use a catheter to urinate for the first couple of days.

During the recovery period, you may experience discomfort, bruising and swelling at the surgical site. It's important to carefully follow the instructions on cleaning and caring for the wound to avoid infections.

Success rates as high as 80 percent have been reported for sphincteroplasty, and about two-thirds of people who have the operation gain substantial benefit. But long-term success rates are lower, 50 percent to 60 percent, particularly when nerve injury is involved. Up to half the people who've had this surgery experience incontinence again, require further surgery or develop other bowel problems.

Even when surgery is successful, you might not have complete bowel control. Your doctor may suggest biofeedback treatment following surgery to help you gain better control of your anal sphincter.

Artificial sphincter

If sphincteroplasty doesn't improve fecal incontinence, or if anal sphincter muscle and nerve damage are extensive — leaving little or no functioning sphincter — a surgeon can create a new sphincter. This is done either by inserting an artificial sphincter or by wrapping a muscle taken from the thigh around the sphincter.

The artificial sphincter consists of three parts — an inflatable cuff that wraps around your anus, a pressure-regulating balloon and a control pump that inflates the cuff. When inflated, the cuff keeps your anal sphincter shut tight until you're ready to defecate. A small tube connects the cuff to the balloon, which is implanted beneath the abdominal muscles. The balloon contains fluid that keeps the cuff inflated.

To go to the bathroom, you use a small external pump to deflate the cuff and allow stool to be released. The pump, which is connected by another small tube to the pressure-regulating balloon, is placed in the labia if you're a woman and in the scrotum if you're a man. When you squeeze the pump, fluid moves out of the cuff into the balloon. After a few minutes the fluid slowly refills the cuff, closing the sphincter.

To avoid problems with wound healing, the cuff isn't inflated until several weeks after surgery. Most people show improvement in bowel control following placement of an artificial sphincter. But the long-term effectiveness is still unknown, and the rate of complications following surgery is high. Infection is the most common and most serious problem, and the device may need to be removed if infection occurs.

Dynamic graciloplasty

Like artificial sphincter surgery, dynamic graciloplasty replaces a damaged anal sphincter muscle. Instead of inserting an artificial sphincter, however, the surgeon uses muscle from another part of the body to substitute for the damaged sphincter. The procedure may be recommended for people with a nonworking sphincter due to muscle or nerve injury.

The name of the surgery comes from the muscle that's transferred — the gracilis muscle, which is in the inner thigh. Occasionally, muscle from the buttocks or forearm is used instead. During the procedure, part of the gracilis muscle is removed and wrapped around the anus, like a sling. Because the transplanted muscle can't be contracted or relaxed, a battery connected by electrodes to the muscle is implanted to control the muscle. This prevents stool from leaking out. When you want to pass stool, you can turn off the electrical stimulation using an external magnetic device.

About 50 percent to 70 percent of people who have this surgery report improvement in bowel control. Like getting an artificial sphincter, dynamic graciloplasty is a major surgery that carries significant risks. Complications can include infection around the electrodes or in the anal or thigh area, muscle detachment or erosion, impaired emptying of the rectum, and battery malfunction.

To avoid exposing your anus to stool while it heals, your surgeon may perform a temporary colostomy or loop ileostomy. A colostomy or ileostomy diverts bowel movements through an opening in your abdomen instead of the rectum. The opening is covered with a special bag to collect the stool. Following recovery from surgery, the colostomy or ileostomy is closed, re-establishing the normal flow of stool.

Sacral nerve stimulation

A promising new treatment for fecal incontinence involves electrical stimulation of the sacral nerves. These nerves run from your spinal cord to muscles in your pelvis. The nerves regulate the sensation and strength of your rectal and anal sphincter muscles. Direct electrical stimulation of the sacral nerves was first shown to be effective in treating urinary incontinence, and studies offer encouragement that it also helps fecal incontinence. (See an image of sacral nerve stimulation on page 91.)

This treatment may be recommended if behavior therapy and medications have failed to improve fecal incontinence, or for people who are still experiencing incontinence after surgery to repair the anal sphincter. Sacral nerve stimulation is most effective if you have an intact anal sphincter.

The procedure is normally done in an operating room at a hospital or outpatient clinic. You'll receive a medication for sedation, as well as a local anesthetic in the involved area — on your backside, below your waist and above where you sit.

Sacral nerve stimulation is done in stages. First the doctor uses an X-ray device to identify the places in the sacrum (the triangular bone in the middle of your pelvis) where the sacral nerves are located. A needle is inserted into the sacral nerves that control the bowel, bladder and pelvic floor. The needle is connected to an external device that generates electrical pulses that stimulate the nerves. The doctor checks muscle and sensory responses to this electrical stimulation.

Once the proper responses have been noted, the permanent (chronic) lead, or wire, is attached to the sacral nerves. The lead is tunneled under the skin and connected to another lead outside the skin. During this initial phase, the electrical stimulation is controlled through a small battery-powered unit that you carry. You'll keep a bowel diary for two weeks to record the results of stimulation. If your incontinence and quality of life improve, you may then return and have the external wire removed and an implantable, programmable battery unit placed under the skin.

The battery unit, or generator, is placed in your upper buttocks and connected to the permanent wire. The unit produces electrical impulses that stimulate the sacral nerves, helping you regain continence. The generator has an external control unit, so you can adjust the programming. You'll also see your doctor every four to six months to make sure the device is programmed correctly. The battery can last five to 10 years.

Sacral nerve stimulation is still considered an experimental treatment for fecal incontinence, but it appears to hold promise. It's much less invasive than other surgical approaches and has other advantages as well. The procedure carries low risks of serious complications and will not worsen symptoms or cause nerve damage.

Other procedures

Depending on the cause of your fecal incontinence and the severity of your symptoms, other surgical procedures may be considered.

Operations to treat rectal prolapse, hemorrhoids and rectocele. Rectal prolapse, a condition in which a portion of your rectum protrudes through your anus, weakens the anal sphincter. In certain circumstances, such as chronic constipation and straining, the ligaments in the rectum can become stretched and lose the ability to hold stool in place. Surgical correction of the rectal prolapse may be needed along with sphincter muscle repair. In women, a protrusion of the rectum through the vagina (rectocele) may need to be treated surgically to correct fecal incontinence. (See images of a normal rectum and vagina and rectocele below.)

Prolapsed internal hemorrhoids can prevent complete closure of the anal sphincter, leading to fecal incontinence. Hemorrhoids may

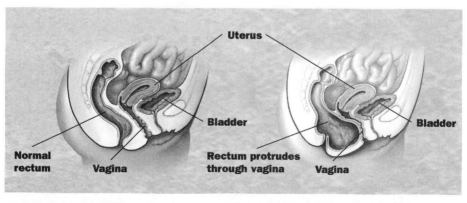

Rectocele is a hernia-like protrusion of part of the rectum into the vagina. Weakened pelvic floor muscles can lead to rectocele and fecal incontinence.

be near the upper part or beginning of the anal canal (internal hemorrhoids) or at the lower portion or anal opening (external hemorrhoids). Hemorrhoids can be treated by conventional hemorrhoidectomy, a surgical procedure to remove the hemorrhoidal tissue.

Colostomy. As a last resort, a colostomy may be the most definitive way to correct fecal incontinence, particularly in older adults. In a colostomy, the surgeon attaches the end of the bowel to an opening in the abdomen. A bag is attached to this opening to collect the stool.

A colostomy can often be performed with minimally invasive laparoscopy, which makes use of a lighted tube (laparoscope) through a small incision. Modern colostomy bags aren't visible when you're dressed, and they control odor very effectively. For many people, a colostomy offers a more socially acceptable alternative to severe, uncontrolled fecal incontinence.

Hope for the future

As you've read, treatment of fecal incontinence depends on its cause. Given the range of treatments available, most people can find some relief. With the right tests and a sensitive, knowledgeable doctor, you can get treatment that offers good results and improves your quality of life.

Appendix

This appendix is a quick reference guide to a variety of tools that can help you and your doctor determine whether you have urinary or fecal incontinence. In addition, it provides lists of medications, foods and beverages that may play a role in your incontinence and offers suggestions of some things you can do at home or work to help reduce the signs and symptoms of incontinence.

Bladder diary

A bladder diary is a detailed, day-to-day account of your symptoms and other information related to urinary habits. It can help you and your doctor determine the causes of bladder control problems.

To keep a bladder diary, simply record what and how much you drink, when you urinate, the amount of urine you produce, whether you had an urge to urinate and the number of incontinence episodes. If you leak urine, note the approximate amount and what you were doing when the leakage occurred. To measure your urine, your doctor may give you a pan that fits over your toilet rim. The pan has markings like a measuring cup. A simpler alternative is to describe the quantity in more general terms, such as small, medium or large. Do what works best for you.

Doctors recommend keeping a bladder diary for two to seven consecutive days and nights. Choose a time that best represents your normal life. Avoid diary keeping during vacations or other changes in routine. In addition, if you're a woman, avoid starting your diary during your menstrual period. Increased trips to the bathroom during this time may skew the findings.

Sample bladder diary

(Make copies of this diary for use in tracking incontinence episodes.)

Time	Fluids		Urinated in toilet (number of times)	How much? (small, medium or large amount)
	What kinds?	How much?		
Sample	*coffee*	*2 cups*	✓	*medium*
6 a.m. to 8 a.m.				
8 a.m. to 10 a.m.				
10 a.m. to noon				
Noon to 2 p.m.				
2 p.m. to 4 p.m.				
4 p.m. to 6 p.m.				
6 p.m. to 8 p.m.				
8 p.m. to 10 p.m.				
10 p.m. to midnight				
Midnight to 2 a.m.				
2 a.m. to 4 a.m.				
4 a.m. to 6 a.m.				

Dietary restrictions

Some of the things you eat or drink may irritate your bladder or bowel and aggravate signs and symptoms of incontinence. By keeping a diary of what you eat and drink and your signs and symptoms, you may begin to see a connection between certain foods and beverages and incontinence. List what you eat and drink, how much you eat and drink, and when you have an incontinent episode.

It's not necessary to avoid all of the items listed on pages 189-191. After you identify a food or beverage that seems to cause problems, try reducing or eliminating that item from your diet for a week or two. If your signs and symptoms improve, consider avoiding the item permanently or at least reducing the quantity you consume.

Bladder irritants
The following list includes foods and beverages that can lead to bladder irritability. Ask your doctor if you have questions about which

Did you feel a strong urge to urinate?	Leaked urine (number of times)	How much? (small, medium or large amount)	Activity when leaking
no	✓ ✓	*small*	*running*

foods or beverages might be causing you problems. Remember that it's not necessary to completely cut out all of the items listed below.

Carbonated beverages
- Soda
- Sparkling water

Alcohol
- Beer
- Wine, wine coolers
- Liquor

Caffeine
- Coffee
- Tea
- Chocolate
- Some medications

Citrus fruits and juices

- Orange
- Grapefruit
- Lemon
- Lime
- Mango
- Pineapple
- Vitamin C supplements

Tomatoes and tomato-based foods

- Tomato juice
- Tomato sauce
- Barbecue sauce
- Chili

Highly spiced foods

- Foods that use chili peppers or other pungent spices (Mexican, Thai, Indian, Cajun)

Milk and milk products

- Cheese
- Yogurt
- Ice cream

Sugar and other sweeteners

- Corn sweeteners
- Honey
- Fructose
- Sucrose
- Lactose

Bowel irritants

Food and beverages that can cause diarrhea and worsen fecal incontinence include:

- Caffeine
- Cured or smoked meats, such as sausage, ham and turkey
- Spicy foods

- Alcohol
- Dairy products
- Fruits such as apples, peaches and pears
- Fatty and greasy foods
- Sweeteners such as sorbitol, xylitol, mannitol and fructose, which are found in diet drinks, sugarless gum and candy, chocolate, and fruit juices

Medications that may cause incontinence

Medications that you're taking for another medical condition may cause or contribute to incontinence. Be sure to tell your doctor about any medications — prescription or over-the-counter, including vitamin and mineral supplements — that you take. If your medication is likely contributing to incontinence, your doctor may be able to suggest a different dose or medication, or a change in the time of day when you take the medication. See charts beginning on page 192 that list medications which may contribute to incontinence.

Pelvic floor exercises

Pelvic floor exercises involve squeezing and relaxing muscles in the pelvic and genital area. These exercises help maintain the strength, endurance and proper action of your pelvic floor muscles, which are important for bladder and bowel control. The exercises are also referred to as Kegel exercises, after Arnold Kegel, the doctor who first described them. When performed correctly, regular pelvic floor exercises can help improve or maintain bladder and bowel control.

How to do pelvic floor exercises

First locate your pelvic floor muscles. Imagine that you're trying to stop from passing gas. Squeeze and lift the rectal area and, if you're a woman, the vaginal area, without tightening your buttocks or belly. You should sense a pulling or closing feeling in your genital area when you squeeze. Men may feel their penis pull in slightly.

Medications that may cause or worsen urinary incontinence

Type of medication	Examples
Water pills (diuretics)	• Furosemide (Lasix) • Chlorothiazide (Diuril) • Indapamide (Lozol) • Spironolactone (Aldactone)
High blood pressure (antihypertensives)	• Prazosin (Minipress) • Terazosin (Hytrin) • Doxazosin (Cardura) • Methyldopa (Aldomet) • Reserpine (Diupres, Diutensen-R, Regroton)
Heart (calcium channel blockers)	• Verapamil (Calan, Isoptin, Verelan) • Nifedipine (Adalat, Procardia) • Diltiazem (Cardizem, Dilacor, Tiazac)
Heart (beta blockers)	• Pindolol (Visken)
Heart (antiarrhythmics)	• Disopyramide (Norpace)
Muscle relaxants and sedatives	• Diazepam (Valium) • Chlordiazepoxide (Librium) • Alprazolam (Xanax) • Lorazepam (Ativan)
Anti-Parkinson's drugs	• Benztropine (Cogentin) • Trihexyphenidyl (Artane)
Anticholinergics (antispasmodics)	• Hyoscyamine (Anaspaz, Cystospaz, Donnamar, Levbid, Levsin) • Oxybutynin (Ditropan)
Narcotic pain relievers	• Morphine • Codeine • Acetaminophen and oxycodone (Percocet) • Oxycodone (Oxycontin)
Cold remedies	• NyQuil • TheraFlu • Alka-Seltzer Plus Cold Medicine • Afrin No Drip
Antihistamines	• Diphenhydramine (Benadryl)

Effect

Overproduction of urine, which may overwhelm an already stressed bladder.

Relaxation of the urethral sphincter, which can lead to leakage of urine.

Relaxation of the bladder muscle (detrusor), leading to incomplete bladder emptying and overflow incontinence.

Relaxation of the bladder muscle, leading to incomplete bladder emptying and overflow incontinence.

Incomplete bladder emptying and overflow incontinence.

Relaxation of the urethral sphincter, leading to leakage of urine. Sedation, delirium or confusion can also diminish awareness of the need to urinate.

Blocked contraction of the bladder muscle. The bladder becomes so full that a sudden, uncontrollable contraction causes overflow incontinence.

Slowed activity in the colon, causing constipation, which may obstruct urine flow and aggravate an overactive bladder.

Slowed passage of food and waste through the digestive tract, resulting in constipation. Constipation can obstruct urine flow and aggravate an overactive bladder.

Incomplete bladder emptying, difficulty urinating, weak stream, leakage, frequency.

Slowed activity in the colon, causing constipation, which may obstruct urine flow and aggravate an overactive bladder.

Medications that may cause or worsen fecal incontinence

Type of medication	Examples
Laxatives and stool softeners	• Methylcellulose (Citrucel), psyllium (Fiberall, Hydrocil, Metamucil, Reguloid) • Magnesium salts (Epsom Salt, Phillips' Milk of Magnesia) • Mineral oil and bisacodyl (FemiLax, Fleet Laxative, Gentle Laxative, Veracolate) • Docusate (DOK, D-S-S)
Anticholinergics (antispasmodics)	• Hyoscyamine (Anaspaz, Cystospaz, Donnamar, Levbid, Levsin) • Oxybutynin (Ditropan)
Antidepressants	• Imipramine (Tofranil) • Amitriptyline (Elavil)
Narcotic pain relievers	• Morphine • Codeine • Acetaminophen and oxycodone (Percocet) • Oxycodone (Oxycontin)
Diabetes medications	• Metformin (Glucophage)
Water pills (diuretics)	• Furosemide (Lasix) • Chlorothiazide (Diuril) • Indapamide (Lozol) • Spironolactone (Aldactone)
Iron and calcium supplements	• Iron (Femiron, Feosol, Feratab, Nu-Iron, Simron) • Calcium (Calci-Chew, Rolaids, Tums)
Antacids	• Maalox, Mylanta, Phillips' Milk of Magnesia, Tu

Here are three ways to practice pelvic floor exercises:
• Holding. This exercise works the muscles' ability to hold. Slowly tighten, lift and draw in the pelvic floor muscles and hold them for a count of three. Relax, then repeat. At first you probably won't be able to tighten the muscles for very long. Start with holding for one to two seconds, and gradually increase over a period of several weeks to a goal

Effect
Diarrhea and urgency.
Slowed activity in the large intestine, causing constipation and possibly fecal incontinence.
Relaxation of the bladder muscle, leading to incomplete bladder emptying and overflow incontinence.
Slowed passage of food and waste through the digestive tract, resulting in constipation.
Chronic diarrhea that may start long after you begin taking the drug.
Increased urine production and loss of salt and water from the body, which can dry stool and lead to constipation.
In some people, constipation or diarrhea.
Drying of the stool, causing constipation.

of 10 seconds. If you feel the contraction letting go, just re-tighten the muscles. Rest for 10 seconds between each contraction. Over time your contractions should also become stronger.

- Quick flicks. This exercise is a series of rapid contractions and releases. You quickly tighten the muscles, lift them up and let them go.

- Urge control. This exercise can be done when you feel an urge to go to the bathroom. First, stop and stand very still. Sit down if you can. Relax. Take a deep breath, then let it out. Try to think of something other than going to the bathroom. Contract your pelvic muscles three to four times to keep from leaking. When you feel the urge lessen somewhat, walk normally to the bathroom. If the urge happens again on the way, stop and repeat the exercise.

You can do pelvic floor muscle exercises almost anywhere — while you're driving, watching television or sitting at your desk. Ask your doctor how many exercises to do each day. One simple starting program is to do 10 before getting out of bed in the morning, 10 after lunch, 10 in the evening while watching television, reading or doing the dishes and another 10 before falling asleep.

After six to 12 weeks of doing pelvic floor exercises correctly, you should notice improvement in your bladder and bowel control. To further strengthen the urinary and pelvic floor muscles, women can use vaginal weights. These are tampon-shaped cones that you insert into your vagina and try to hold in place. You'll know you're doing the contraction incorrectly if the cone falls out. As your contraction technique improves and your muscles grow stronger, you increase the weight of the cone.

Things to remember
A few key things to remember when doing pelvic floor exercises:

- Avoid doing them while urinating. This can cause difficulties in emptying your bladder.
- Don't strain as you're doing these exercises. Your abdominal, buttock and thigh muscles shouldn't tighten. Put your hand on your belly. If your hands feel pressure, you're straining.
- To double-check that you're contracting the right muscles, try the exercises in front of a mirror. Another way to be sure you're doing the exercises correctly is a simple finger test. Place a clean finger in your anus or vagina (for women). This may be easier to do while you're in the shower or with the help of a rubber glove and a lubricant such as K-Y Jelly. Then squeeze around your finger. The muscles you contract are

your pelvic floor muscles. If you're still not sure if you're using the right muscles, ask your doctor to refer you to a physical therapist for biofeedback techniques that will help you identify and contract the right muscles. Electrical stimulation is another alternative.

- Although you may not be able to hold the contraction for more than a second at first, with regular practice you'll be able to hold your contractions longer.
- Contract your pelvic floor muscles *before* an event that causes you to leak urine, such as nose blowing, sneezing or coughing. For example, as you feel the urge to cough, tighten your pelvic floor muscles before and during your cough.
- After the first few days of doing the exercises, you may notice some soreness around your pelvic area. This is normal and will ease as your muscles become stronger. But don't overdo it. If the soreness becomes too uncomfortable, talk to your doctor.

Bowel diary

A bowel diary is often used along with a record of what you eat and drink to help determine the cause of fecal incontinence. In a bowel diary, you record the date and time of your bowel movements, the consistency of the stool, whether you felt the urge to go and any incontinence episodes. It's also helpful to note any feelings of straining, discomfort or incomplete emptying, and use of enemas or laxatives.

Doctors recommend keeping a bowel diary for at least one week. Choose a time that best represents your normal life. Avoid diary-keeping during vacations or when there are other changes in your normal routine.

Use the bowel diary beginning on the next page to keep a record of episodes of fecal incontinence. You may want to make copies of the diary and keep them in the bathroom to make it easier to record each episode. Keeping a bowel diary can be an important first step in determining the cause of your incontinence.

Sample bowel diary

Record one bowel episode per column of the diary, even if there is more than one a day. Choose the best answer for each question. Copy diary as needed.

Date: _____	Date: _____
Time: _____ a.m./p.m.	Time: _____ a.m./p.m.
Amount of stool ☐ None ☐ Staining ☐ Minor soiling ☐ Major soiling	☐ None ☐ Staining ☐ Minor soiling ☐ Major soiling
Did you have to hurry to the toilet? ☐ Y ☐ N	☐ Y ☐ N
How long did you hold your bowel movement?	Minutes:
Stool description (Circle the number below that best describes consistency.)* 1 2 3 4 5 6 7	1 2 3 4 5 6 7
Did the episode occur while you were sleeping, or did it wake you from sleep? ☐ While sleeping ☐ Woke me	☐ While sleeping ☐ Woke me

*Stool consistency: pellets = 1, formed and hard = 2, formed and soft = 3, semiformed = 4, mushy = 5, loose = 6, watery = 7

Bladder drills

Bladder drills (timed-voiding exercises) are a form of bladder training, or urinating on schedule. The goal is to improve urinary continence by gradually:

- Increasing the length of time between your trips to the bathroom
- Increasing the amount of fluid your bladder can hold
- Decreasing the sense of urgency and leakage you experience

The changes in your urinary habits take place over 12 days or so. It's best to start on a weekend or a day when you plan to be home or near a bathroom. You may want to talk to your doctor before starting this plan.

When following this program, consider the following tips:

- Make sure to drink enough fluid every day. Drinking appropriate amounts and emptying your bladder at regular intervals helps decrease the risk of bladder infections.

Date: _____
Time: _____ a.m./p.m.

☐ None   ☐ Staining
☐ Minor soiling ☐ Major soiling

☐ Y   ☐ N

Minutes:

1 2 3 4 5 6 7

☐ While sleeping
☐ Woke me

Date: _____
Time: _____ a.m./p.m.

☐ None   ☐ Staining
☐ Minor soiling ☐ Major soiling

☐ Y   ☐ N

Minutes:

1 2 3 4 5 6 7

☐ While sleeping
☐ Woke me

- Keep a bladder diary (see pages 188-189) as a way to track your progress.
- You're the best judge of how quickly you should advance to the next step. These guidelines are general suggestions, but you may find that a different pace works better for you. For example, you might decide to increase the time between voidings every two days instead of every three. Or you may find it more comfortable to move from urinating every hour to every $1^1/4$ hours instead of $1^1/2$ hours.
- When you feel a sense of urgency to go before the next scheduled time, try doing pelvic floor muscle exercises (see page 191). If possible, sit down until the sensation passes. Remind yourself that your bladder isn't really full, and try to think about something else.
- Over several weeks or months, you may find that you can wait 3 to $3^1/2$ hours between trips to the bathroom and that you have fewer feelings of urgency and episodes of incontinence.

Bladder drill schedule

Days 1 to 3	After waking up, empty your bladder every hour on the hour, even if you don't feel the need to go. Make sure you're drinking at least eight glasses of fluid each day. During the night, only go to the bathroom if you wake up and have to go.
Days 4 to 6	Increase the time between emptying your bladder to every 1½ hours, with the same fluid and night instructions as above.
Days 7 to 9	Increase the time between emptying your bladder to every two hours, with the same fluid and night instructions as above.
Days 10 to 12	Increase the time between emptying your bladder to every 2½ hours, with the same fluid and night instructions as above. Work up to urinating every 3 to 3½ hours.

Questions for your doctor

To find a doctor to help with incontinence, start by asking some questions. Once you have a short list of possible care providers, call their offices. Or you could make an appointment to interview the doctor to see how he or she communicates with you. One of the most important things a doctor can do is to acknowledge your problem with sympathy and support.

Following are some possible questions to think about when choosing a doctor:

- What is the doctor's education and training regarding incontinence?
- How long is the wait for an appointment?
- Is the doctor part of your health insurance plan?
- Does the doctor listen to your concerns about incontinence, answer your questions and explain things clearly?
- Does he or she seem sincerely interested in treating incontinence?

Once you've chosen a care provider, you may have questions about medications, tests and treatment.

About tests:
- What will this test show?
- How accurate is it?
- Are there any risks or side effects?
- Will it be uncomfortable?
- Do I need to do anything special before or after the test?

About medications:
- Why do I need this medication?
- Are there any side effects?
- How soon should my symptoms improve?
- Are there any special instructions?

About treatments:
- What are the benefits and risks?
- When can I expect to see improvement in my condition?
- Are other treatments available?
- Can you refer me to another doctor for a second opinion?
- If surgery is needed, how long will I be hospitalized?
- What's the average recovery time?
- Can my condition be cured?
- What incontinence and skin care products would help me manage better?

Incontinence symptoms questionnaires

To determine the severity of your symptoms, your doctor may ask you to fill out a questionnaire about your experience with incontinence. Several different symptom questionnaires — sometimes called quality of life assessments — have been developed for both urinary and fecal incontinence. These questionnaires serve as tools to help your doctor assess the severity of symptoms, make treatment decisions and evaluate the success of various approaches to treatment. The questionnaires also can help you and your doctor understand how incontinence is affecting your overall quality of life.

Some more commonly used quality of life questionnaires used for urinary incontinence include the Incontinence Impact Questionnaire (IIQ), the Urogenital Distress Inventory (UDI), and the International Prostate Symptom Score (IPSS) — for men.

Additional resources

The AGS Foundation for Health in Aging
The American Geriatrics Society
www.healthinaging.org

Alliance for Aging Research
2021 K St., N.W.
Suite 305
Washington, D.C. 20006
(202) 293-2856
www.agingresearch.org

American Foundation for Urologic Disease
1000 Corporate Blvd.
Suite 410
Linthicum, MD 21090
(800) 828-7866 or (410) 689-3990
www.afud.org

American Medical Women's Association
801 N. Fairfax St.
Suite 400
Alexandria, VA 22314
(703) 838-0500
www.amwa-doc.org

American Urogynecologic Society
2025 M St., N.W.
Suite 800
Washington, D.C. 20036
(202) 367-1167
www.augs.org

American Urological Association
UrologyHealth.Org
www.urologyhealth.org

Bladder Advisory Council of the American Foundation for Urologic Disease
www.incontinence.org/index

International Continence Society
9 Portland Square
Bristol BS2 8ST
United Kingdom
44-117-9444881
www.continet.org

International Foundation for Functional Gastrointestinal Disorders (IFFGD)
P.O. Box 170864
Milwaukee, WI 53217
(414) 964-1799 or (888) 964-2001
www.iffgd.org

National Association For Continence (NAFC)
P.O. Box 1019
Charleston, SC 29402
(800) 252-3337 or (843) 377-0900
www.nafc.org

National Digestive Diseases Information Clearinghouse (NDDIC)
2 Information Way
Bethesda, MD 20892
(800) 891-5389
www.digestive.niddk.nih.gov

National Institute on Aging
Building 31, Room 5C27
31 Center Drive, MSC 2292
Bethesda, MD 20892
(301) 496-1752
www.nia.nih.gov

National Institutes of Health
9000 Rockville Pike
Bethesda, MD 20892
(301) 496-4000
www.health.nih.gov

National Kidney and Urologic Diseases Information Clearinghouse (NKUDIC)
3 Information Way
Bethesda, MD 20892
(800) 891-5390 or (301) 654-4415
www.kidney.niddk.nih.gov

National Women's Health Information Center
8550 Arlington Blvd.
Suite 300
Fairfax, VA 22031
(800) 994-9662
www.4woman.gov

The Simon Foundation for Continence
P.O. Box 815
Wilmette, IL 60091
(800) 237-4666
www.simonfoundation.org

Index